THE 6-PACK CHECKLIST

A STEP-BY-STEP GUIDE TO SHREDDED ABS

BY: NATE MIYAKI
www.NateMiyaki.com

Copyright © 2015 Nate Miyaki

Published by **Archangel Ink**

ISBN: 1516975553
ISBN-13: 978-1516975556

Table of Contents

SECTION 1: INTRO & BIGGER PICTURE STRATEGIES 1

Get Back to the Basics 2

The People's 6-Pack Champ 5

Focus on Your Diet First 10

SECTION 2: THE OFFICIAL 6-PACK CHECKLIST 15

Step #1—Get in the Calorie Deficit Necessary for Fat Loss 16

Step #2—Reduce Refined & Hyperpalatable Foods 24

Step #3—Emphasize High-Satiety Whole Foods 32

Step #4—Eat Adequate Protein 39

Step #5—Strength Train to Maintain Lean Muscle 44

Step #6—Moderate Your Dietary Fat Intake 53

Step #7—Adjust Your Carbs as Necessary 63

Step #8—Ditch the Fitness Myths & Find a Sustainable Diet Structure 72

Step #9—Add NEPA if Necessary 84

Step #10—Track Your Food Intake if You're Having Trouble 89

Step #11—Make Subtle Adjustments at Sticking Points 94

Step #12—Integrate Carb Refeeds When Lean 97

SECTION 3: OUTRO 107

6-Pack Checklist Summary 108

The Final Fat-Slashing Strategy 110

Thank You 111

Please Leave a Short Review 112

Other Books by Nate Miyaki 113

Resources 114

About the Author 117

SECTION I
INTRO & BIGGER PICTURE STRATEGIES

Get Back to the Basics

> *Nothing fancy is involved. You go straight to the heart of the matter and defeat the enemy. There is nothing else involved. You either do it or you don't.*
> —Miyamoto Musashi

Everyone seems to be chasing after a lean body and a glorious 6-pack these days—you, me, and the great Nacho Libre. But most people are running down the wrong roads, dead-end streets, or paths with too many pitfalls. Thus, they are failing to reach their final, belly fat–free destination.

Maybe you know what that frustration feels like and are looking for a better way to reach your elite physique goals.

Here is the tough-love truth: fat loss success rates suck. They barely stand at a sickly 2-20%, depending on the studies and statistics you use. Success is defined as the ability to lose body fat AND keep it off for more than a year.

Crash diets followed by rebounds and constant yo-yo-ing don't count. Neither does popping in some "extreme training" video and jumping around like a cheerleader on crack for 90 days, then recovering from all of your injuries or burn out on the couch the rest of the year.

And surprisingly enough, alternating between a 6-pack "in-season" and looking 6-months pregnant in the off-season probably doesn't count either. Jumping from jagged-edge cuts to jiggly-wigglies just doesn't jive with the fact that objective fat loss numbers never lie.

There is no doubt about it, Man Boobs & Muffin Tops are tenacious tag team opponents that are hard to keep down for the count these days. We're a long way away from our really, really, ridiculously vain goals of living lean year-round.

Fundamental Strategies & Steps vs. Get Fit Quick Tricks

There are a variety of reasons for this staggering lack of fat-slashing success. Perhaps the biggest is that in the Internet era, we've gotten way too caught up in chasing after magic pills, quick fixes, and cutting edge trends. We are too easily distracted by biohacks, insider tricks, and minutia that doesn't really matter that much in the end.

"Click this ad to learn the one weird trick fitness models use to get shredded." Well, I've worked as a fitness model a few times, and I can tell you the only "weird" thing is that people still believe that BS exists.

Tricks are for kids, and portly ones at that. Trust me, I know. They used to call me the Baby Sumo & Boob (because I was a little ball of fat that everyone liked to squeeze). But they're not for adults who are trying to build a board short- or bikini-ready body and don't believe in fat loss fairy dust.

As a result of this scatterbrained attack, we have lost our ability to focus on the basic fat loss steps. We have moved too far away from the fundamentals that produce 95% of real-world results.

To be honest, it is not just the general public that has been led astray. Many athletes, trainers, authors, and fitness bloggers have gotten bit by the overcomplication and quick-fix syndromes, and are suffering the side effects of that toxic venom. So if you just choose some random program or diet, your chances of finding success with your higher-level physique goals are slim (pun intended).

If you would rather streamline and simplify your physique transformation plan and implement a practical approach that produces consistent results, then you need to take care of the highest-level fat loss steps first.

You need to hack away the unessential and focus on just a few basic, proven strategies so that when either the ridiculousness of the fitness industry or your own emotion or lack of patience tries to take you on a detour, you have the right road map to stay on the most productive path.

I hope this book filters through the fitness industry fluff, brings those key fat-loss fundamentals back into the forefront of your mind, and gives you the step-by-step plan you'll need succeed with your goals.

If you start at the top of the hierarchy of importance (step #1), work your way down the list, and check things off one by one (as you apply them, NOT just read about them), you will surely find the way to shed your body fat disguise and unveil the 6-pack gift that anatomy has bestowed upon all of us.

The People's 6-Pack Champ

Why am I 100% confident I can help you finally reach your higher-level fat loss, physique transformation, and shredded 6-pack goals?

Is it my formal credentials in the Sports Nutrition, Personal Training, or Exercise Science fields? Not really. Who gives a damn about scientific pontification and paper credentials?

Well I do, and you probably should too. But that stuff is pretty boring to start with, and I need to better grab your attention right off the bat somehow, lest you go off and buy some other fitness book that leaves you spinning your wheels with strategies that sound good on paper but don't actually produce results in the real world.

I'd say given the specific, shallow topic at hand, I have to go a little douche bag on you to start. I apologize in advance for that very questionable play call.

Practical "Pack" Experience

Here's what you really need to know. I've had a 6-pack for the last dozen years or so. Yep, that's right. Unlike a lot of fitness professionals, I actually follow the advice that I write about and have practical experience with the strategies I speak of. Here is a current, non-professional, non-photoshopped photo:

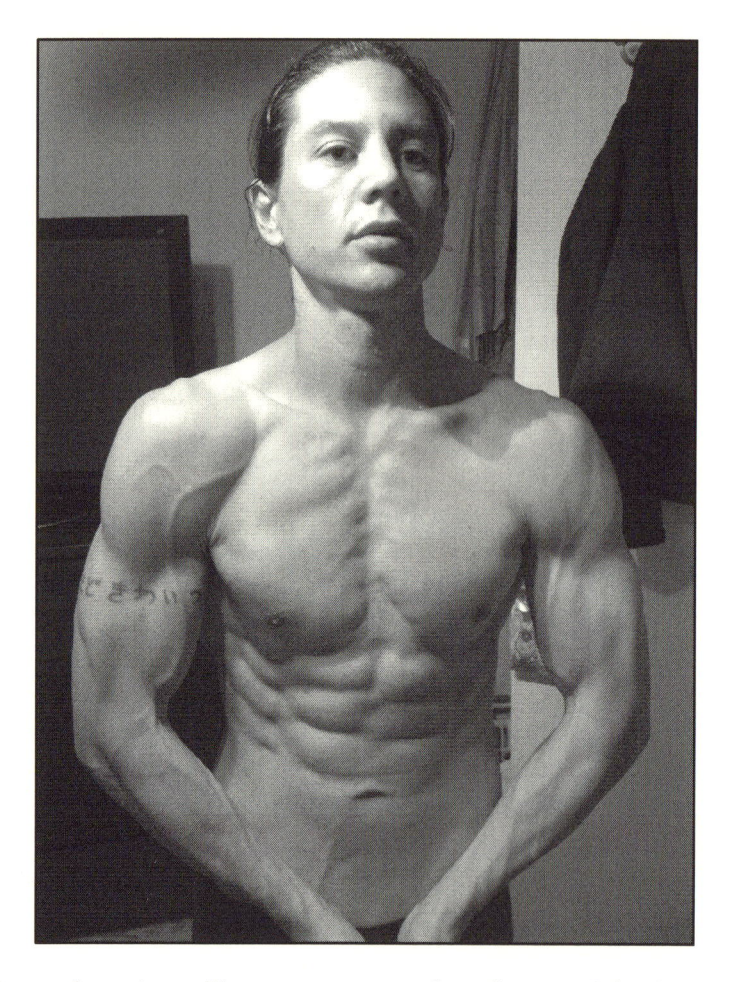

Over that time, I've won a couple of natural bodybuilding competitions, represented some fitness brands, and have even been paid to take off my clothes as a fitness model a few times. I'm not very "equipped" below the belt, if you dig what I'm saying . . . so the cash was solely for the 6-package above it.

Again, I am sorry for dropping that douchebagness on you. It's just that the fitness industry is full of frickin' frauds these days. Most people have no clue how to get and STAY ripped, and this includes most "fitness professionals" who write the articles and ads about their self-proclaimed, insider 6-pack secrets.

There are no secrets, baby. There are only straightforward, physiologically based strategies. You either follow them and ultimately find your way, or you don't and keep wasting time chasing magic 6-pack pixie dust.

Wow, in just a few short paragraphs, I'm already sick of myself, so let's get to the REAL reasons why I believe I can help you.

Perhaps the most important qualification is that I've managed to help plenty of other people reach their peak physique goals. I guess that's why I'm known worldwide—or at the very least, in my own mind—as The People's 6-Pack Champ.

You can check out what The People have to say here: natemiyaki.com/testimonials

Or maybe you prefer a video montage with mostly half-naked people (and my actual formal credentials). Here you go! youtu.be/ILZOIH7EJSQ

Your 6-Pack Success Story

But this book isn't about me. Nor is it about the physique peeps I've worked with in the past. This book is about you. I want you to get out there with an informed plan in hand, take action, and write your own 6-pack success story.

I believe I can teach you a step-by-step physique transformation process that works in the real world, not just one that sounds good on paper, in magazines, at nutrition conferences, or in fitness forums.

I've written about some of these strategies in magazines like *Men's Fitness, Muscle & Fitness, T-Nation,* and Bodybuilding.com.

My goal with this specific book is to put all of those strategies into one place, hack away the unessential, and narrow it down into a simple checklist that you can follow in order to slash body fat and carve out a 6-pack.

I hope we can fulfill that mission together.

P.S. A 6-Pack Won't Change Your Life

Do you think a 6-pack will bring you fortune? As I said, I've done several professional fitness model shoots and been in some of the mainstream magazines, and the pay is crap.

Do you think a 6-pack will bring you fame? Unless you like Borat-style high-fives from the dude working out next to you at the gym, who always smells like beef and cheese (sometimes with a hint of onion), no one in the real world really cares about your 6-pack except you. Trust me on that one.

Do you think a 6-pack will make you happy? Not to get too philosophical on you, but happiness is an internal thing, not an external one. It is about passion, self-actualization, and living up to your own core values, not anyone else's. It is about digging yourself, not depending on the approval of anyone else.

> *Care about people's approval and you will be their prisoner.*
> –Tao Te Ching

> *The more you value things, the less you value yourself. The more you depend upon others for esteem, the less you are self-sufficient . . . Freedom discovers man the moment he loses concern over what impression he is making or about to make.*
> –Bruce Lee

So make sure you are starting this process for the right reasons, else it will fizzle just as quickly. And I don't want to be the dude selling you modern guru snake oil.

But perhaps you just want to challenge yourself to see how good of shape you can actually get in. There are other ways—more physique-focused ways—to do that other than running a marathon.

Maybe just going through a process that requires some education, effort, consistency, discipline, determination, delayed gratification, patience, and perseverance can positively affect other areas of your life.

Or maybe it's just because 6-packs are a pretty awesome thing from an aesthetic perspective, and you want to rock one on a regular basis.

Just don't think achieving some superficial goal is somehow going to change your life.

Finally, I don't care what any modern "movement," corrective exercise expert, or functional training guru says; 6-packs are absolutely functional. If you are stuck with a small piece below the belt line like me, you can't have a big ol' belly and still get the job done in the bedroom. The physics of it all just doesn't work out.

So depending on the size of your shiitake, you just might have no other choice but to shed that belly fat down to a 6-pack in order to perform optimally in the sack. And, baby, it's debatable whether moving like an animal is all that "functional." But mating like one absolutely is.

Alright then, my friend, enough of the poops and pontification, the sh!znits and giggles! Let's get this thing rolling (or more accurately, let's get that body fat rolling off your body!).

Focus on Your Diet First

> *"Body sculpting is 85% diet . . . if you don't have your diet down first, the rest is moot . . . People are often skeptical of my statement that bodybuilding is 85 percent nutrition. The average bodybuilder vastly underestimates the value of diet and overestimates how good his own eating program is."*
> –Vince Gironda

This is more of a big picture, theoretical thing than an actual practical step, so I'm including it here vs. in the step-by-step strategies. But I think it is absolutely critical to understand before we get started with our plan.

If you retain only one piece of information from this book, or any of my past or future content, I hope that it's this: your nutritional habits will have a far greater impact on your fat loss and 6-pack goals than any other fitness component.

If you've read any of my past books, you've heard this principle before, but sometimes you have to sound like a broken record to finally break through.

Offline, I work primarily as a trainer, yet I always start with that statement first.

Sure, there are some outliers with great genetics who can eat whatever they want and look great. But for most of us with average genetics—definitely me, and probably including you—just can't out-train a crappy diet.

How can I lose fat the quickest? Clean up your diet.

What is the best exercise for 6-pack abs? Load up a backpack full of the packaged food in your cabinet, walk down to your nearest homeless shelter, and give it to some people who need it more.

Give me the fat loss secret, Nate. No problem, my friends. Stop looking for magic pills and start improving your daily nutrition habits. See what I'm saying?

My Experience as a Physique Athlete & Fitness Coach

I've been in the fitness industry for fifteen years now, have personally trained hundreds of people, and have advised thousands more. I've worked with pro athletes, entertainers, natural bodybuilders, bikini girls, fitness models, busy professionals, start-up entrepreneurs, doctors, delivery truck drivers, high-level investors, stay-at-home moms, strippers, and crazy people alike.

There has been only one universal theme.

The clients who used diet as their primary weapon in the war on fat loss were the ones who obtained the best results. They won—swiftly and efficiently.

The clients who tried to use exercise to offset a poor diet, or who thought they could eat whatever they wanted because they were exercising, obtained mediocre results at best. They tried to out-train a poor diet. They are still fighting a battle they will never win.

I learned this lesson the hard way myself. There was a time in my life where I was a good performance athlete—sprinter, martial artist, acrobat, and stunt performer. I did this all while being skinny-fat.

It wasn't until I nailed down my diet that I was able to attain a lean physique and gain some success in the fitness world.

Real-World Fat Loss Examples

If you look around your gym, you've probably noticed some regulars who have been there day in and day out for months, or even years, but look exactly the same. How can there be all of that time and effort with no results to show for it? The answer is diet, of course, or lack thereof.

Another good example is professional NFL offensive linemen. These guys are pro athletes who perform vigorous training protocols on a daily basis. They are big, strong, fast, and could certainly throw me a severe beating. Most of them, however, have a little jiggle with their wiggle. A large percentage of them are obese.

How can it be that there are world-class athletes who are fat? Again, the answer is poor or no nutritional strategy.

Even most "fitness experts" these days will have to hire fitness models to promote their products. You'd be surprised how many trainers pumping products or authors writing magazine articles about revolutionary training programs are OUT OF SHAPE! What's the reason?

Again, they may have the best training programs in the world, but their diet sucks.

Conversely, when you hear tales of dramatic weight loss or great body transformations, nutrition is always at the forefront of the discussion. "How did you lose the weight?" friends will ask. "Oh, I went on such and such diet" or "I read this or that nutrition book."

Was that book *The Truth about Carbs* by any chance (shameless book plug alert)?

Or was it Jared and his "6-incher"? But seriously, people can make drastic changes in their physique with diet alone.

And where do you stand? Can you squat and bench heavy loads but are also carrying an extra load around the waist? Can you perform amazing boot camp and cross-training drills but don't look like you've ever exercised a day in your life? Can you hit amazing running times but are still soft, saggy, and flabby crossing the finish line?

Please keep the following in mind so you stop wasting time—the rules for improving performance are different than those for changing appearance.

Why Diet is Often Overlooked

If diet sits atop the fat loss hierarchy, why is it so often overlooked? Here are a few reasons:

1. What sounds better from a marketing standpoint? We have the revolutionary new Navy Seal-like workout that is going to kick your a$$ and get you ripped vs. dude or girl, you gotta stop eating so much crap?

   The former does, of course, especially if you have a slice of pizza in your hand while watching that infomercial. But despite what looks good in an ad, the reality is the latter is what is really going to get you noticeable results. It is less sexy, but it is way more effective.

2. You CAN perform well on a crappy diet. There is no arguing that from some of the diet logs I've looked at in my lifetime. So you may be lifting heavy and getting stronger or getting better at your running times or totals, performing cross-training drills, etc., but are you looking the way you want or should, given all of that hardcore training you've been doing—shredded, ripped, lean, tone, tight, or whatever?

3. Sure, you may be able get away with whatever you want nutritionally in your 20s, but the small percentage who maintain a lean physique into their later years are the ones who took care of their bodies and followed an informed path right from the beginning.

   Don't wake up in your 30s, 40s, or 50s saying, "I'm doing everything I used to do, but I'm out of shape now." It's because what you were doing from the beginning wasn't the right way.

4. And crazy fitness chicks, if you have to do two hours of cardio a day, twice a day, plus metabolic circuits every hour, on the hour, plus down fat-burning pills like Peanut M&M's, etc., to get lean now, what are you going to do in your 40s?

The Cutting Conclusion

Well, my fat loss friend, I'm rambling on, as always. The main moral of the story is that you can't change your body just by exercising. As a matter of fact, I'd say the majority of you—if your goal is getting a lean, beach-ready physique—are wasting your time in the gym until you clean up your diet and implement a sound nutrition protocol.

Until you make some changes in your diet, any training program—even the greatest training program in the world, or the revolutionary new one, or the program with all of those lost training "secrets"—will be meaningless.

If you are stubborn and still think you are going to outrun a poor diet, or that your training program is so "hardcore" you can eat crap all day, then stop reading right now. I can't help you. Come back when you are actually ready to get your 6-pack.

Miyaki's Preferred Method: Use Diet as Your Primary Fat Loss Weapon

The simple summary of my fat-slashing style, so far: Use diet for 80% of your fat loss.

SECTION II
THE OFFICIAL 6-PACK CHECKLIST

Step #1—Get in the Calorie Deficit Necessary for Fat Loss

Step back from the scientific pontification and diet industry debate about whether or not calories matter and think about carving out a Greek God- or Goddess-like 6-pack from an objective perspective.

How many people do you know who say something like, "Calories don't count; you only need to worry about carbs, kale, caveman foods, detoxing, drinking more water, or whatever the latest hot diet topic is . . ." are actually as lean as you'd like to be?

That's why you see most of them wearing sweaters in webinars rather than walking around with their shirts off, pants off, or rolling around naked (hey now!).

Sitting around and sounding like you know what you are talking about is a hell of a lot easier than proving you know what you are doing by getting into elite shape in the real world.

Now flip the script. How many physique athletes and fitness models do you think know their calorie intake down to the last decimal point? And if you are tracking the grams of your macros—protein, carbs, fats—you are indirectly tracking calories.

You must ask yourself an important question right now, my friend. Which is more important to you: sounding like you know what you are talking about when it comes to 6-packs or actually getting one? Those routes are very different.

If it's the latter, then let's get something straight right off the bat, baby. Calories definitely matter and are the most important number to get right in the fat loss equation. They are not the only number, as many calorie-counting diets proclaim, but they are the most important one.

The Calorie Deficit vs. The Composition of the Diet

> *Each year many people go on a diet to lose weight. An active area of research is examining the efficacy and safety of energy-deficient diets that have different proportions of the macronutrients. At this time size of the caloric deficit appears to be more important to weight loss than the composition of the diet. Weight loss has been reported with both low-carbohydrate, high-fat diets and high-carbohydrate, low-fat diets.*
> –Gropper et al. Advanced Nutrition and Human Metabolism

Despite some of the metabolic and hormonal advantages of certain foods and macronutrient ratios, total calories are still king. The only way to force your body to burn off stored fat is to take in fewer calories than you expend, on average, over some time frame.

Yes, certain foods—higher protein, not necessarily low carbs—offer a metabolic advantage (a higher percentage of calories are burned off in the digestion process), have greater impacts on satiety, and are less likely to be overeaten and stored as body fat.

Certain macronutrient amounts and ratios can impact blood sugar, satiety, insulin, glucagon, growth hormone, cAMP, HSL, and other hormones and enzymes that control fat storing and fat burning processes.

This is why you see so many diet books focused on how "protein is powerful" or "cutting carbs is cool." The nerd in me can't deny that these scientific processes are dead sexy. There is nothing like a frickin' biochemistry lecture to get your girl or dude in the mood, right??

But if you want to go all the way and seal the deal (wait, what are we talking about here? Living lean year-round or getting laid . . . or both?), the bottom line remains: attaining an average negative energy balance is the most important step for fat loss.

And to be honest, this whole "Calories vs. Metabolic Advantage Debate" (if you don't know what I'm talking about, I envy you for having a balanced life outside of fitness) is all really a useless circle-jerk debate anyway. If you want to get into elite shape, everything matters—calories, macronutrient amounts and ratios, the metabolic and hormonal impacts of foods, your ratio of gym time to personal mirror reflection time, etc.

And don't worry. You don't need to run out and get a PhD to get into elite shape. Although the technical science behind the fat loss process is crazy complex and could take a lifetime to learn, the actual "what to do" in the real world is straightforward and simple. And you'll automatically be covering it all as you work your way down our checklist.

The Misunderstood Macro-Calorie Connection

Even if you are a "macronutrient" guy or gal (e.g., you gotta go low-carb to get lean), when you cut out a certain macronutrient, you are automatically cutting calories. If you are lowering your carb intake, you're lowering overall calories—four calories per gram of carb you cut.

On the flipside, if you are lowering your fat intake, you are lowering overall calories—nine calories per gram of fat you cut.

If you are improving your food quality by going Paleo or vegan or all-natural or whatever (the actual philosophical reason for removing refined food is irrelevant), chances are that change led to a reduction in total calories—1500 calories or so for every supersized Meal #5 you cut out.

In all of the above scenarios, you were cutting calories whether you were conscious of it and counting or not.

Now, those are all scenarios where ignoring calories can still go right. Let's talk about some scenarios where it can go wrong.

What happens when people just focus on macronutrients and forget about the most important step in the fat loss hierarchy?

Low-Fat Diets in Caloric Excess

Well, we learned some valuable lessons from the low-fat era of the 70s, 80s, and 90s. First, feathered and hair-sprayed hair is totally cool and will never go out of style. I don't care what modern hipsters and fashionistas say.

Second, you can cut your fat intake to zero, but if you are eating above your total calorie limits with low-fat cereals, snack packs, and sugar bombs all day, a bunch of bad things can happen:

1. Once liver glycogen is full, and once muscle glycogen is full, the excess carbs will be stored as fat.
2. With excess fuel and chronically elevated blood sugar and insulin levels, the body has no need to burn fat as a fuel source. The body will never be forced to tap into its internal body fat stores as a reserve fuel (you won't lose any body fat). It will just be trying to burn through all of that excess sugar all day—kind of like a kid in a candy store running around like a chicken with its head cut off.
3. In addition, any dietary fat you take in will not get used as an immediate fuel source. It will simply be stored as fat (you will gain body fat).

Low-Carb Diets in Caloric Excess

What happens when you go low-carb but still overeat total calories?

Many modern low-carbers and Paleo proponents are making the exact same "messing with the macronutrients before tackling total calories" mistake. It's like Jason & Friday the No-Fat 13th vs. Freddie Krueger & A Nightmare on No-Carb Street.

They are both horror stories, just with different slashing styles (or in our case, the inability to actually slash fat).

You can cut your carbs to zero, but if you are eating above your total calorie limits via unlimited dietary fat intake (downing butter and bacon bombs all day, pouring cream and oil over every meal like a gangster paying tribute to his homies, etc.), here are some things to consider:

1. Lowering carbs and insulin increases fat oxidation (fat burning) rates. But increased fat oxidation rates do not necessarily equal lower body fat, no matter how intelligent or cool the word sounds.
2. If you are in a state of caloric excess and there are fatty acids constantly circulating in your bloodstream from an unlimited dietary fat intake, your body will use those ingested fats as energy first BEFORE tapping into body fat stores.
3. If you are eating above your total calorie limits, there is no physiological reason for your body to break down body fat. That's an unnecessary extra step, and your body prefers the most efficient route to energy production possible, despite you wishing for something different.
4. Forget the boring technical terms. The bottom line is that it doesn't matter if your body is a "fat-burning machine" if you are only burning ingested dietary fats instead of body fat. You won't lose the love handles and get lean.
5. Quite the opposite is true. Excess calories will be stored as body fat regardless.

You don't have to memorize the boring biochemistry of either situation. Just remember this: total calories determine where your fuel is coming from (ingested food or internal body fat) and the ultimate fate of that fuel (burned off vs. stored).

Or, excess calories equals extra body fat, no matter how you slice up your macronutrient pie.

So even if you go low fat, you still need to pay attention to the amount of carbohydrates you are taking in (in order to control overall calories) if you want to get lean.

And even if you go low carb, you still need to pay attention to the amount of dietary fat you are taking in if you want to fulfill your 6-pack dream.

Why We Try to Skip the Calorie Step

Why do we cling to low-carb, low-fat, or low-common-sense diets while trying to dismiss total calories?

"Macro-bashing" plays to our desires. It demonizes a certain macronutrient and points to it as the cause of all of our body fat problems. Eliminate that nutrient, and you can eat as much as you want of everything else.

That's what we really want to hear, isn't it? You can eat as much of "X and Y" as you want, as long as you don't eat "Z."

Sure, eat all of that cheese, ice cream, oil, butter, and bacon as long as you don't have that carb gram from a carrot stick.

Or eat all of those low-fat, processed snack foods, smoothies, and sugary desserts as long as you don't eat any saturated fat from good ol' steak and eggs, etc.

In a world of overindulgence, we want to be able to gorge on something. It doesn't work that way. Controlling total calories is the unfortunate fat loss truth. You can keep wasting time trying to get around that, or you can take the most efficient, straight-line path to slashing fat.

Calorie Cutting Options

I don't want to be a total Debbie Downer and the bearer of all bad news, because I'm a generally happy beach dude who likes to bring a little joy into the life of anyone he interacts with. So as my dear friend the Joker once said, "Let's put a smile on that face."

The good news is that once you are in a calorie deficit, a wide variety of diet approaches can work for fat loss and physique enhancement—typical bodybuilding and fitness programs, Paleo and caveman plans, vegetarian and vegan adventures, if-it-fits-your-macronutrient maestros, cultural and common sense diets, etc.

So you can ultimately find what resonates and works for you vs. getting suckered into the battle for diet supremacy. I certainly have my preferred route that I'm going to share with you in this book (physique-style numbers + island-style diets). But I'd be lying to you if I said a variety of other approaches don't work well either.

And honestly, I don't care how you get the calorie-cutting job done, as long as you do it. If you don't want to track your food intake or count your calories, and focusing on improving food quality is the more feasible way to get you in the deficit necessary for fat loss, I'm all for it.

This is the foundation of several diets—Paleo, raw, whole foods, etc. Specific food templates are used to get you to avoid certain foods (mostly modern, processed, refined foods) and emphasize better ones (mostly real, whole, natural foods—this can range from near-carnivore to near-vegetarian).

For some, this approach works great. The improvement in food quality automatically leads to a reduction in calories. Fat is lost. Abs are found. Beautiful.

For others, this strict food choice approach is too restrictive. Making a wholesale change in their typical meals and food choices is too big of a leap. They struggle with adherence and alternate between "being good" and breaking protocol and bingeing.

Sometimes the slide lasts for weeks, months, or becomes their baseline plan because "fat loss dieting is too strict and unrealistic." Their plan is to just grow the Buddha belly so big that they can ultimately wish it away.

For this group, the easiest and most seamless place to get started is to try to get in a calorie deficit with the foods they are already eating. If you want to go this route, it will mean tracking your food intake and numbers, and adjusting the portion sizes as necessary to get in a deficit.

This approach can definitely work in the short-term. But I'll tell you why I don't think that is the best solution for a long-term, sustainable plan in the next section.

Please never forget the flipside to this fun and flexible calorie story. If you are "eating healthy" or "low-fat" or "going Paleo" or "going raw" but are still not losing weight, shedding flab, and getting lean, now you know why:

Despite eating according to any dogma's creed or false promises, if you're not in a calorie deficit, you won't slash fat and unveil your 6-pack—plain and simple.

Miyaki's Preferred Method: Use Some Simple Fat-Slashing Starting Points

How many calories should you shoot for as a starting assessment point?

There are more complex formulas (Harris-Benedict, Katch-McArdle, etc.), but all numbers must be adjusted and refined anyway based on real-world progress and feedback. And to be honest, I think most of those textbook formulas overestimate how many calories people really need to get lean.

So here are a few simpler, ballpark starting assessment points:

1. If you are sedentary, or only perform low-intensity activity (walking, low-intensity versions of yoga, etc.), start at ten calories per pound of lean body mass. If you don't know your lean body mass, use your target bodyweight.

   But don't expect to get a 6-pack if you are sedentary. If you are severely overweight and deconditioned, you can use this approach to lose a significant amount of weight in the beginning. But eventually, you are going to have to earn your higher-level goal of building a beach body with some kind of higher-intensity exercise.

2. If you are moderately active—you perform one to three moderate to high-intensity training sessions per week (running, biking, strength training, cross-training, performance-based sports, more vigorous forms of yoga, bar-hopping, tantric sex, etc.)—start at 11 calories per pound of lean body mass. If you don't know your lean body mass, use your target bodyweight.

3. If you are very active—four or more moderate-to-high-intensity training sessions per week—start at 12-13 calories per pound of lean body mass. If you don't know your lean body mass, use your target bodyweight.

Step #2—Reduce Refined & Hyperpalatable Foods

I hope the key takeaway from the last section stuck. We can argue over optimum dietary approaches into eternity—Paleo vs. vegan, avoiding sugar vs. eating spinach, juicing vs. jambalaya, etc.

But consistently hitting targeted numbers will always be the most important step in achieving ANY higher-level physique goal—fat loss, muscle gain, body recomposition, total body transformation, etc.

You can set, assess, adjust, and refine the diet numbers to achieve virtually any physique goal you desire. That's why we started our fat loss conversation with the mind numbing details of calorie deficits—it's the most important number to get right.

There is real truth to pure calorie counting and IIFYM (if it fits your macros) diets. If you don't know what the second one is, it's basically a more detailed version of calorie counting and factors in the importance of your macronutrient amounts and ratios as well (like adequate protein levels for preserving lean muscle mass, which we'll talk about in a future section).

The overall theory is that as long as you hit the right amounts of your calories, protein, carb, and dietary fat levels, you can eat whatever foods you want and reach your weight loss goals. In other words, make whatever foods you want to eat fit your targeted diet numbers, and you're good to go.

Many bodybuilders, bikini divas, fitness models, and twenty-somethings follow this approach with great success. And it may just work for you too.

But, and I mean a big ol' "it's all about the bass" butt . . .

There are a few outliers with great genetics and super-fast metabolisms who can eat whatever they want, burn it off, and look great. But for most of us with average genetics and metabolic rates, it is extremely difficult to stay in that calorie deficit necessary for maximal fat loss for any meaningful length of time if you are eating a bunch of processed, refined, or hyperpalatable foods.

The Problems with Refined & Hyperpalatable Foods

> *Many researchers believe that these industrial foods are contributing to the obesity epidemic . . . A common view is that industrial foods promote obesity because they are "hyperpalatable": so palatable that people will continue eating them even after they are full . . . Food reward, not hunger, is the main driving force behind eating in the modern obesogenic environment. Palatable foods, generally calorie-dense and rich in sugar/fat, are thus readily overconsumed despite the resulting health consequences . . . These findings collectively suggest that obesity can arise when animals or humans are confronted with foods whose palatability/reward value greatly exceeds that to which they are genetically adapted.*
> –Paul Jaminet

Here's the real, fat-slashing deal. Any diet plan can work for the short-term when motivation is high—say for an upcoming athletic event, for beach season, or just for updating your e-dating site profile or Facebook page. Most plans focus on this quick-fix mentality.

However, it is virtually impossible to stay in the relative calorie deficit necessary for fat loss, at least for any meaningful length of time, if you are making mostly poor food choices.

Or, put another way, the foods that are making the average population overweight are the same foods that are difficult to diet on for advanced athletes during calorie deficits geared towards maximum fat loss. You just can't cut calories while eating mostly crap and expect to stay the course.

This is where point systems or other calorie-counting diets fail. This is also where I've seen extreme IIFYM approaches fail. You're not going to be able to stay on a reduced-calorie diet plan for long eating pop tarts, low-fat snack packs, and TV dinners.

Fake foods like this are just empty calories with no functional nutrients. They have no effect on satiety or the hormones that regulate appetite and energy intake. You will feel constantly hungry, deprived, and miserable dieting on these foods. In other words, you will constantly feel like you are DIEting.

That's why people yo-yo on and off these plans. They are not sustainable. And it's not because YOU went off the diet. It's because THE DIET was not sustainable in the first place.

Motivation can make any plan work in the short term, even less than ideal ones. That's how motivation works. But it eventually wears out, and thus, doesn't make things automatic.

And that's where we ultimately want to get to for our goal to seamlessly stick: 6-pack automation. We want a year-round lean physique, not just a single weekend a year one.

Food Reward, Hunger Control, & Mindless Eating

I think most of us know 64 oz sodas, supersized fast food #5s, a whole pizza pie, boxes of packaged snack foods, and King Kong–size desserts aren't good for us. Some of this is obvious, but some of this operates on a more subconscious level that most of us just aren't aware of.

That's why we continue to eat these foods on a regular basis even though we know how bad they are for our overall health and wellness and, more important, for our specific physique goals.

In other words, cutting back on these detrimental foods goes beyond just sheer discipline and willpower, because those resources are limited and unpredictable.

It's about education, awareness, avoiding mindless eating for the most part, and implementing some targeted strategies throughout the very tough transition period. It's about working hard to break bad habits, starting some better ones, and then riding the wave of momentum once they are established. It's not always easy in the beginning, but it does get easier if you can power through initially.

The two main problems with refined and hyperpalatable foods are:

1. Hyperpalatable foods override the natural hunger and satiety controls in our bodies (and more specifically, the brain). In the modern world with unlimited access to hyperprocessed and hyperpalatable foods, most of us are eating much more for food reward rather than real physiological need. This leads to chronic caloric excess and body fat gain.

2. There are scientists hired by processed food companies to create the most palatable foods possible. They experiment with different combinations of refined sugar, fats, salt, and flavorings to make these foods almost impossible to not overeat. You can't avoid them, and you can't stop eating them once you start. I won't go as far as to say they cause addiction, but they operate on similar pathways. Food companies are literally exploiting natural food reward mechanisms in the human body to increase their sales (and, unfortunately, our waistlines in the process).

The bottom line is that if you think you are going to be able to moderate your portions of these foods on a regular basis in order to drop body fat, I think you are sadly mistaken.

What Are the Most Hyperpalatable & Easily Overeaten Foods?

> *What are the most highly rewarding foods? Generally speaking, modern processed foods are the most "rewarding"—typically in a combination of refined sugars and fats, mixed with artificial flavorings that are professionally engineered to maximize the reward factor in the brain . . . If a large portion of your diet consists of these foods, you are likely to get dysfunction in the appetite regulation center of your brain and have serious issues with chronic overeating.*
> –Ari Whitten, author *The Low Carb Myth*

The obvious one is refined sugar. We just eat way too much of that sh!znit. It's not necessarily that sugar is a toxic food (although in ultra-high amounts it can be, metabolically).

Sugar is so damn easy to overeat (especially combined with refined flour and refined fats) that it has sent our average calorie intake through the roof, and thus, our body fat levels bursting through the seams.

If you're basically drinking coffee ice cream in liquid form every morning (caramel mochas) and combining it with a sugar-loaded pastry, you're going to have a hard time slashing fat and carving out a 6-pack.

Now that's not to let refined fats off the hook and say that low-carb, unlimited fat diets are the best way to go for shedding fat. In fact, I think it is quite the opposite. I think we've come full circle in the nutritional world to where those are even more problematic and are the primary reason why the modern health and physique-conscious crowd (living in our low-carb era) is failing to reach their final fat loss destination.

Get this: consumption of refined salad dressings and cooking oils has increased a whopping 1450% over the last century! This is how you get supposedly "healthy" gourmet meals and salads that actually contain 1500 calories or more.

Remember, you gotta get in a calorie deficit if you want to get ripped. And it is very hard to do that if you are eating a diet high in refined sugar OR refined fat. Combine the two and you can, as Donnie Brasco said, "forget about it."

How many Health & Wellness Hippies and No-Carb Hipsters do you know who are actually in elite shape?

These results have indicated that the size of an eating episode is influenced by the level of hunger and the nutrient composition of the foods consumed. High-fat foods (probably due to higher energy density) lead to a passive overconsumption which generates a relatively weak satiety.

Green et al. 1994. **Effect of fat- and sucrose-containing foods on the size of eating episodes and energy intake in lean males; potential for causing overconsumption.** *Eur J Clin Nutr* Aug;48(8):547-55.

The Cafeteria Diet Example

As I said above, it's not just a carb or fat thing. It's a crappy refined food thing. We just eat way too much of it these days. Honestly, I don't think people even realize that refined foods make us eat so much more than we are meant to eat or physiologically need.

Here is an analysis by obesity researcher Stephan Guyenet on a study regarding what was referred to as "the Cafeteria Diet." This may put this topic into the proper perspective for you. Numbers never lie . . .

The first study was published in 1992, and seems initially to have simply been an attempt to design a novel way of accurately measuring food intake in free-living humans, which is notoriously difficult. Investigators created an "automated food-selection system" consisting of two large vending machines filled with a variety of prepared foods of known calorie and nutrient compositions. They recruited ten lean, healthy men. At the beginning of the experiment, the investigators took four days to determine each volunteer's energy requirement for weight maintenance.

Then, in the setting of a metabolic ward where no other food was available, the volunteers were allowed to select and eat as much food as they pleased from the vending machines over seven days. The foods available included English muffins, French toast, pancakes with syrup, scrambled eggs, chicken pie, cheeseburgers, margarine, white sugar, various cakes and puddings, apples, jelly beans, Doritos, M and M's, apple juice, 2% milk, sodas and several other foods.

I doubt the investigators were prepared for what they observed when they turned the ten men loose on those vending machines. They immediately began consuming excessive calories, an average of 1,544 kcal per day in excess of their previously determined energy needs (with a fairly typical macronutrient composition by percentage). That amounts to a roughly 60% increase in calorie intake over baseline, a striking change, particularly since it was completely voluntary. Over the course of seven days, the volunteers gained an average of 5.1 lb (2.3 kg).

Larson et al. **Spontaneous overfeeding with a 'cafeteria diet' in men: effects on 24-hour energy expenditure and substrate oxidation.** Int J Obes Relat Metab Disord. 1995 May;19(5):331-7.

Again, the italicized analysis was by Stephan Guyenet. I highly recommend you read his work on food reward, hyperpalatability, non-industrialized cultural diets, and obesity research in general on his blog: Whole Health Source.

Here are a couple of specific articles to start with:

1. The full Cafeteria Diet Study Analysis:
   http://bit.ly/1HndhVl
2. The Case for the Food Reward Hypothesis of Obesity Series: http://bit.ly/1SErGbC

Miyaki's Preferred Method: Cut Back on the Crap to Start Slashing Fat

Let's summarize what we've covered so far.

1. If you want to slash fat and unveil a 6-pack, you have to get in a calorie deficit.
2. If you want to make getting into, and staying in, that calorie deficit as easy and sustainable as possible (so you can stay lean year-round, not just suffer for a short-term goal), your

best bet is to cut back on highly refined, processed, and hyperpalatable foods.
3. This includes refined carbs (sugar, flour, etc.) AND refined fats (oils, butter, creams, sauces, etc.), AND especially fast and packaged foods that combine them both (processed snack foods, pastries, desserts, etc.). Notice I said cut back, not completely eliminate. We'll talk about sustainability strategies in future sections.
4. Instead, make real, whole, natural foods the foundation of your fat-slashing approach.
5. Or, in other words, before you start worrying about carbs vs. fats or any of that other crap, think about improving your ratio of real to refined foods.

Step #3—Emphasize High-Satiety Whole Foods

> *Eat a diet comprised completely (or almost completely) of whole, unprocessed foods. This simple step will to a large degree eliminate highly rewarding processed food from your diet, and will allow you to get back into harmony with eating because of biological need, not because you're trying to give yourself pleasure. This is the essential principle of a good fat-loss diet . . . Whole, unprocessed food allows the amount of fullness you feel while eating to be in tune with how many calories you actually ate. In other words, by eating whole foods you will feel "full" and stop eating sooner than you will with processed foods. This means you will eat enough to be content while eating less.*
> *–Ari Whitten*

More so than the over-the-top marketing material of "miracle foods," I believe the real magic of high quality food choices when it comes to fat loss is that they improve the calorie-to-nutrient density ratio of the diet and also improve satiety, which makes staying in the calorie deficit necessary for fat loss a whole hell of a lot easier.

Ease of plan equals long-term adherence. And long-term adherence is the only thing that equals the real-world success that seems to be so elusive these days.

It's easier to stay faithful to your fat loss plan when it emphasizes real, whole, natural, juicy melons (or long bananas, whatever you prefer) . . . I mean food.

As an experiment, I've had female clients struggle to net 1200 calories a day and male clients 1800 calories a day when they cut out all refined foods (including oils) and ate only real foods.

You don't have to go to that extreme, but the lesson is that it is much easier to stay in the calorie deficit necessary for fat loss, while still giving your body all of the essential nutrients and micronutrients it needs, indefinitely, if you are at least emphasizing real, whole, natural foods.

With certain food choices, you will be much more prepared to make your 6-pack stand, even in the modern food environment with more enemies trying to invade your belly fat stores than the ancient Persian armies.

Different Diet Templates That Automatically Reduce Caloric Intake

Now this may all sound like theoretical mumbo jumbo so far, but there is actually real research out there that validates these claims:

METHODS: Twenty-nine male ischemic heart disease patients with impaired glucose tolerance or diabetes type 2 and waist circumference > 94 cm, were randomized to ad libitum consumption of a Paleolithic diet (n = 14) based on lean meat, fish, fruit, vegetables, root vegetables, eggs, and nuts, or a Mediterranean-like diet (n = 15) based on whole grains, low-fat dairy products, vegetables, fruit, fish, and oils and margarines during 12 weeks. . . .

RESULTS: The Paleolithic group were as satiated as the Mediterranean group but consumed less energy per day (5.8 MJ/day vs. 7.6 MJ/day, Paleolithic vs. Mediterranean, $p = 0.04$). Consequently, the quotients of mean change in satiety during meal and mean consumed energy from food and drink were higher in the Paleolithic group ($p = 0.03$). Also, there was a strong trend for greater Satiety Quotient for energy in the Paleolithic group (p = 0.057).

CONCLUSIONS: A Paleolithic diet is more satiating per calorie than a Mediterranean-like diet.

Jonsson et al. **A paleolithic diet is more satiating per calorie than a mediterranean-like diet in individuals with ischemic heart disease.** Nutr Metab (Lond). 2010 Nov 30;7:85.

In his analysis and interpretation of the above study, obesity researcher Stephan Guyenet made some additional points:

Despite receiving no instruction to reduce calorie intake, the Paleolithic group only ate 1,388 calories per day, compared to 1,823 calories per day for the Mediterranean group. That's a remarkably low ad libitum calorie intake in the former (and a fairly low intake in the latter as well).

With such a low calorie intake over 12 weeks, you might think the Paleolithic group was starving. Fortunately, the authors had the foresight to measure satiety, or fullness, in both groups during the intervention. They found that satiety was almost identical in the two groups, despite the 24% lower calorie intake of the Paleolithic group.

In other words, the Paleolithic group was just as full as the Mediterranean group, despite a considerably lower intake of calories. This implies to me that the body fat 'set point' decreased, allowing a reduced calorie intake while body fat stores were burned to make up the calorie deficit.

Now, here is the real crazy thing about this study. It is comparing two relatively healthy diet approaches, and there is still a significant difference when it comes to satiety and auto-regulating a reduced calorie intake.

What do you think happens when we compare either approach to a typical Y2K highly refined, processed, and fast food diet? Well, remember the Cafeteria Diet from the last section?

The average ad libitum calorie intake (eat as much food as you want based on hunger) on the Cafeteria Diet was 4550 calories per day. The average ad libitum calorie intake on the Mediterranean Diet was 1823 calories. The average ad libitum calorie intake on the Paleolithic-style diet was 1388 calories.

So you see, while a calorie deficit is definitely the most important fat loss step, food choices factor in in terms of auto-regulating that reduction in calories. Or, good food choices make getting into the calorie deficit necessary for higher-level fat loss a hell of a lot easier, all while ensuring higher nutrient density and lower hunger. This, in turn, makes that approach a hell of a lot more sustainable. Hell yeah!

What Are the Highest Satiety Foods?

What are the highest satiety foods you can emphasize if you want to keep hunger under control during your fat-slashing diet? Well, the above research study pretty much summed it up.

Additional research confirms the highest satiety foods are root vegetables (potatoes, sweet potatoes, yams), whole fruit, and animal proteins. So much for low-carb diets being the most sane and sustainable way to slash fat. I'd say the bet with the best odds of succeeding on your fat loss quest is a diet low in refined foods and high in whole foods.

Of course, it should come as no surprise that the low-satiety foods you should cut back on are processed foods full of refined sugar, vegetable oil, and/or flour.

Satiety Index Chart

FOOD	RANKING
High Satiety Foods	
Boiled potatoes	323%
Fish	225%
Oranges	202%
Apples	197%
Beef	176%
Eggs	150%
Low Satiety Foods	
Yogurt	88%
Peanuts	84%
Candy Bar	70%
Doughnuts	68%
Cake	65%
Croissant	47%

Holt et al. **A satiety index of common foods.** Eur J Clin Nutr. 1995 Sep;49(9):675-90.

Translating Research into Real-World Templates

Sometimes it is good to get outside of the fitness world full of ads for protein shakes, sports drinks, meal replacements, and magic fat-burning pills and look at healthy cultural diets for real, unbiased clues about what to eat for optimal health and efficient fat loss.

Common food staples among some of the healthiest and fittest cultures in the world, ones that don't even really focus on "dieting" per se (Okinawan, Kitavan, Traditional Japanese, Traditional Hawaiian, etc.), seem to include fish, meats, wild game, eggs, vegetables, starchy root vegetables (sweet potatoes, potatoes, taro), rice, and whole fruit (including higher fat fruits like coconut and avocado).

Those sound exactly like the ones at the top of the satiety index chart, huh?

A Little Leeway for a Lifestyle Plan

If you are eating high quality food 85-90% of the time, you can include some crap while still losing significant amounts of body fat.

So what I recommend doing is making healthy island-style meals your foundation (eggs and fruit, steak and potato, fish and rice, chicken and sweet potato, all with some optional non-starchy vegetables in unlimited amounts), and then including a few cheat meals a week (usually on the weekend when you are out socializing and don't want to be limited or stressed about your diet).

That's a lot more doable as a long-term lifestyle plan than trying to cut out the foods you love indefinitely. A little bit of flexibility right from the beginning yields a lot more long-term sustainability.

But the key is the ratio of quality-to-crap. It doesn't have to be 100-0 as some militant diet cults and dogmatic creeds proclaim. But it can't be 30-70 like it is for most of us these days living post-Y2K. We need to toughen up and improve upon that ratio in order to slash fat and look awesome.

Miyaki's Preferred Method: Eat an Island-Style Diet

When you combine all of the above info from this chapter and the last and translate that into a practical template you can keep in the back of your mind for simplicity's sake, you get what I have come to call an island-style diet approach.

It's like a Paleo/caveman-style diet with a few more starchy carbs from root vegetables and rice in order to better fuel and recover from the high-intensity training that is going to be necessary to build muscle, slash fat, and carve up your 6-pack.

1. Animal proteins—fish, shellfish, poultry, meat, game meat, eggs.
2. Whole fruit—juicy melons, long bananas, perfect peach bottoms, strawberries in the sack . . . whatever you prefer. Also berries, pineapple, apples, oranges, etc.
3. Root vegetables (also called starchy tubers = the geekiest word on the planet)—yams, sweet potatoes, potatoes, taro root, burdock, pumpkin, squash, etc.
4. Vegetables—you know, greens 'n' things.
5. White rice—this is a special case with a long, boring, and geeky story behind it. The short summary is that white rice is a pure starch without all of the compounds in most cereal grains that can be problematic for human digestion, and it can be included as an additional carb source in the diet once your baseline essential nutrient and micronutrient needs have been met by animal and plant foods. For more on this topic, you can read <u>this post</u> on my website.

I think an island-style diet is one of the healthiest and most delicious ways to live lean year-round. But I'm just a beach dude married to an island girl, so maybe I'm biased as hell as well . .

Step #4—Eat Adequate Protein

So far, we've talked about:
1. Getting in a calorie deficit
2. Reducing refined and hyperpalatable foods
3. Emphasizing high satiety whole foods

Once you are in a calorie deficit and emphasizing high quality whole food choices, there are a variety of macronutrient (protein, carbs, fats) distributions and ratios that can work well for fat loss.

Low-carb, high-protein, and near-carnivore plans can work. Just keep in mind that there is a big difference between eating high-quality meat, fish, eggs, coconut, etc. within the confines of a calorie deficit vs. eating low-quality processed meats, fried foods, and oils in unlimited amounts.

High-carb, low-fat, near-vegan diets can work as well. Just keep in mind that there is a big difference between eating high-quality whole fruits and root vegetables within the confines of a calorie deficit vs. emphasizing crappy processed foods like vegan muffins, cookies, smoothies, and pizza in unlimited amounts.

But if optimizing body composition is your goal—getting lean while maintaining your lean muscle mass and shape (vs. just skinny or skinny-fat)—one of the things I definitely recommend you do is to eat a decent amount of protein.

Protein & Lean Muscle Preservation

Adequate protein (along with strength training) helps us preserve lean muscle mass while staying in the calorie deficit necessary for fat loss. This is critical, as lean muscle is what provides our body with its shape, tightness, tone, and definition. Thin, soft, flabby, and lots of jiggling with your wiggling is not the look we're after.

So despite being in a calorie deficit to drop fat, we want to eat the right amount of protein to support our lean muscle mass. In other words, protein is not just for the meatheads trying to sell tickets to their gun shows. It is for the divas trying to drop the muffin tops, too.

Fitness and Sports Nutrition is geared towards crazy people . . . I mean individuals engaging in a regular exercise program. This means your protein needs are likely higher than the RDA recommendations for two reasons:

1. The RDAs are set for the general, non-exercising population. Exercising, especially weight training, places unique stresses on the body. The constant breaking down and rebuilding of muscle tissue increases the body's demands for protein.
2. The RDAs are set to avoid the side effects related to protein deficiency and for maintenance of the average physique, not for the higher aspirations of meatheads and divas looking to maximize lean muscle mass while stripping away body fat.

Protein-Based Meals and Satiety

As we already talked about in the last section, protein is one of the highest satiety foods. So it makes good sense to base most of your main meals around a high-quality protein source to control hunger during a fat loss diet.

Research confirms the effectiveness of this strategy.

Eating fewer, regular-sized meals with higher amounts of lean protein can make one feel more full than eating smaller, more frequent meals, according to new research from Purdue University. We found that when eating high amounts of protein, men who were trying to lose weight felt fuller throughout the day; they also experienced a reduction in late-night desire to eat and had fewer thoughts of food.

We also found that despite the common trend of eating smaller, more frequent meals, eating frequency had relatively no beneficial impact on appetite control. The larger meals led to reductions in appetite, and people felt full. We want to emphasize though that these three larger meals were restricted in calories and reflected appropriate portion sizes to be effective in weight loss. Our advice for people trying to lose weight is to add a moderate amount of protein at three regular meals a day to help appetite control and the feeling of fullness.

Leidy HJ et al. **Influence of higher protein intake and greater eating frequency on appetite control in overweight and obese men.** Obesity (Silver Spring). 2010 Mar 25.

Don't Follow Bodybuilding Extremes

Protein should be the foundation of your diet, but it should not be excessively high as many extreme bodybuilders, hardcore muscle magazines, and protein supplement companies recommend.

Steroids increase protein synthesis, and those using them may indeed be able to utilize excessively high amounts of protein for supra-physiological processes. This is not true for the natural athlete or regular exerciser.

In high amounts, especially combined with low-carb diets, a process called deamination occurs where the body strips amino acids of their nitrogen molecule and converts them to glucose. This is a metabolically (and literally) costly way to obtain glucose.

Forget the boring biochemistry. This just means that although the athlete's goal is to fuel their muscles first, your body's evolutionary goal is to fuel the brain first. Your body will find a way to fuel the brain before anything else, even if it means breaking down protein, or even your own muscle tissue, to do so. I know it might not seem like it if you've ever had a conversation with a full-blown meathead or diva, but it's the physiological truth.

When excess dietary protein is converted to glucose, the body must excrete the remaining nitrogen through the urine (the scientific term is pee-pee). And although high-protein diets don't cause kidney disease, excessively high protein intakes do force the kidneys to work harder than is necessary.

And at some point, despite what many proclaim about unlimited protein diets, there can be drawbacks. At very high amounts (5+g/kg), you can exceed the liver's capacity to convert excess nitrogen to urea and excrete it through the urine. This causes blood ammonia levels to rise, which can lead to gastrointestinal distress and general fatigue.

If you are interested in this topic, I recommend you check out the following paper. I've included a few key highlights to wet your protein knowledge appetite.

1. The accepted level of protein requirement of $0.8g \cdot kg^{-1} \cdot d^{-1}$ is based on structural requirements and ignores the use of protein for energy metabolism. High-protein diets on the other hand advocate excessive levels of protein intake on the order of 200 to 400 g/d, which can equate to levels of approximately $5 g \cdot kg^{-1} \cdot d^{-1}$, which may exceed the liver's capacity to convert excess nitrogen to urea. Dangers of excessive protein, defined as when protein constitutes > 35% of total energy intake, include hyperaminoacidemia, hyperammonemia, hyperinsulinemia, nausea, diarrhea, and even death (the "rabbit starvation syndrome").

2. The key issues are the rate at which the gastrointestinal tract can absorb amino acids from dietary proteins (1.3 to 10 g/h) and the liver's capacity to deaminate proteins and produce urea for excretion of excess nitrogen.

3. This gives us an initial understanding that although higher protein intakes are physiologically possible and tolerable by the human body, they may not be functionally optimal

in terms of building and preserving body protein. The general, although incorrect, consensus among athletes and bodybuilders is that rapid protein absorption corresponds to greater muscle building.

Bilsborough et al. A Review of Issues of Dietary Protein Intake in Humans.

Research on Optimum Protein Amounts

So we need more than the RDA but less than the steroid extreme. What's the sweet spot?

The majority of the research suggests 1.5-2.0g/kg, which equals 0.7-0.9g/lbs of bodyweight.

Although there remains some debate, recent evidence suggests that dietary protein need increases with rigorous physical exercise. Those involved in strength training might need to consume as much as 1.6 to 1.7 g protein x kg(-1) x day(-1) (approximately twice the current RDA).—The International Journal of Sports Nutrition

For SA (strength athlete), the LP diet (low protein 0.9g/kg) did not provide adequate protein and resulted in an accommodated state (decreased WBPS [whole-body protein synthesis vs. MP and HP]), and the MP (moderate protein—1.4g/kg) diet resulted in a state of adaptation (increase in WBPS and no change in leucine oxidation). The HP diet (high protein 2.4g/kg) did not result in increased WBPS compared with the MP diet, but leucine oxidation did increase significantly, indicating a nutrient overload.— The Journal of Applied Physiology

Miyaki's Preferred Method: A Moderate Protein Diet Foundation

Shoot for a daily protein intake of 0.7-0.9g/lbs of lean body mass or target body weight (if you want, you can round up to the fitness standard of 1g/lbs of lean body mass for a little extra satiety and muscle preserving insurance).

For my metric friends, this equals 1.5-2.0g/kg of lean body mass or target body weight (rounding up to 2.2g/kg of lean body mass if preferred).

Step #5—Strength Train to Maintain Lean Muscle

The foundation of our efficient fat-slashing approach is starting to take shape:

1. Get in a calorie deficit
2. Reduce refined and hyperpalatable foods
3. Emphasize high satiety whole foods
4. Eat an adequate amount of protein

At this point, we need to take a quick detour into the training realm because, the truth is, you are not going to maintain muscle and improve the shape and tightness of your body just by eating protein. That would be pretty awesome, though, if that were the case.

Protein simply provides us with the raw ingredients necessary to build lean muscle. You need to actually send a physical signal to your body to spark that physiological process.

Damn, that sounded too geeky. Let's rephrase—you actually have to earn your 6-pack and muscle shape with some exercise.

How do you best do that? Enter Sandman? Nope. Enter the Dragon? Nope. Enter strength training.

The Big Physique Transformation Picture

We should take a step back for a second and talk about my overall approach to the fat loss and physique transformation process.

After close to 20 years in the game, here is what I have found to be the fastest, most effective, most efficient, and most sustainable way to transform your physique and look good at the beach (at least for a busy professional who wants to maintain some sort of career, family, social, and sex life).

1. Use diet for 80% of your fat loss.
2. Strength train to build lean muscle & shape, tighten, and tone your body.
3. Increase non-formal activity levels (i.e., walk more as part of your day) for the final 20% of fat loss.

Don't Waste Your Time Training to Burn Fat

If diet gives you 80% of your fat loss results, and a little increase in non-formal activity levels gives you the final 20%, why would you spend a bunch of time trying to burn fat when you exercise? The answer is you shouldn't, at least if you want the most efficient path to results possible.

So why should we exercise at all? Exercise can preserve lean muscle while dieting, or ensure a greater percentage of weight lost is coming from body fat, not lean muscle mass.

If pure physique transformation is your goal, when you hit the gym, you should be trying to build muscle—period. Muscle is what provides your body with its shape, definition, tone, and tightness. Strength training is far superior in this respect to cardiovascular exercise and should be the focus of your exercise routine.

Diet alone can definitely help you lose weight, but if you're skinny with NO muscle tone (because you have lost a bunch of lean muscle mass throughout that weight loss process), you will still appear loose, flabby, soft, and unimpressive, despite a low body weight.

That's not quite the type of beach body you had envisioned for yourself. So you could say that strength training to maintain muscle—while your diet takes care of the majority of fat loss—doesn't just "pump the body up." It can keep it "tight like a tiger" (*Goldmember*), too.

If a shredded 6-pack is your goal, don't just watch the scale. Look in the mirror (or at photos). Lean muscle is equally as important as low body fat.

Think of our physique transformation path as a two-pronged approach. You want to minimize body fat and maximize lean muscle mass (yes, you too, ladies). As we already said, diet is your primary weapon to slash body fat.

Exercise should be your primary weapon to build lean muscle mass.

Basic Strength Training vs. Cardio & Cross-Training

What about all of those plans marketed as the best "fat-burning" workouts—cardio-based programs, running, boot camp and cross-training drills, etc.? They are all really helping you improve PERFORMANCE. You build up muscular and cardiovascular endurance and get better at performing the specific drills, etc.

If your sport requires those skills or physiological demands, or you just enjoy that style of training, then that's exactly the type of program you should be following.

But my philosophy is you will more efficiently improve your APPEARANCE by using your diet to burn off most body fat and using your formal exercise sessions to focus on basic strength training in order to build lean muscle.

Women & Weights

Muscle growth is a healthy process that provides many physical benefits. Too often, people (frequently women) do not engage in resistance training because they are afraid it will make them "too big." This unfounded fear can prevent them from obtaining the full benefits of a strength-training program. Not only do women have fewer muscle fibers than men, especially in the upper body, but additionally, the primary anabolic (muscle-building) hormone—testosterone—is dramatically lower in women than in men. Therefore, women rarely develop overly large (or "manly") muscles without the use of anabolic drugs. With a well-designed resistance training program, women typically see an increase in the muscle size with a corresponding decrease in body fat, resulting in smaller dimensions and improved muscle definition.—National Strength & Conditioning Association

I have no doubt that combining a solid diet with a targeted strength training routine is the fastest way to attain a flat belly and a bikini-ready body. But many women shy away from lifting weights for fear of bulking up.

The real explanation for the difference in bulking up and looking masculine between men and women is a difference in hormone levels. Men have higher amounts of testosterone, a highly anabolic hormone that leads to increased muscular growth. Women have higher levels of estrogen, which leads to more body fat accumulation and is the reason why women, on average, carry more body fat than men.

Women have miniscule amounts of testosterone compared to men, and their propensity to bulk up from weight training is very limited compared to that of a man. By the way, the overly masculine female bodybuilders you sometimes see in magazines are injecting themselves with steroids (synthetic versions of the male hormone testosterone) in order to attain unnatural levels of muscularity. Unless you are "juicing" it up, you have no reason to fear you'll morph into the Incredible Hulk.

This also means, however, that women must work even harder than men to build lean muscle, increase their resting metabolism, and get lean. I've seen several couples begin a body fat reduction program at the exact same time. With all things being equal (training, diet, adherence to the two), the man always gets results faster than the woman because of these testosterone/estrogen differences.

Women, you have to work twice as hard as a man to get half of the results. It is not fair, but it's the genetic truth. And in the end, it's worth it. Muscle is denser than body fat. A lean, firm, sculpted triceps takes up less space and appears less "bulky" than a triceps covered in body fat (turkey arms syndrome). Which would you prefer?

Stick to Basic Bodyweight & Free Weight Exercises

Much of the fitness industry has it backwards. The gym is full of complicated, wild, and new exercises and exercise systems backed by little scientific basis. It's all about the trends and the fads and what sells (products or services), not about what is truly effective.

Efficient training for physique development is exactly the opposite of the fitness trends and fads. It uses the complicated science of Kinesiology and Biomechanics to yield relatively simple exercises and simple programs.

Now don't misunderstand me. That means simple on paper, but it is actually challenging in its implementation and execution.

With all of the complexities of the human body, human movement really comes down to nothing more than a simple lever system. Attach some resistance onto the end of that lever (i.e., a dumbbell) and you have yourself a results-producing exercise.

It's not rocket science, it's physics, and the actual real world application is simple common sense.

You don't need crazy, weird exercises that have you balancing on balls, twisting, and flipping all over the place, unless you are training specifically for those performance needs (I used to train that way for stunt performances, by the way).

You need simple movements that overload the muscles and provide the initial spark for the adaptation process. That's how you efficiently build a body. The basics may not be cool or hip or innovative or cutting edge, but they damn sure are effective!

"Old-school," basic exercises get bashed in the modern fitness industry as unintelligent and uninformed. I will concede that many juiced-up meatheads and pill-popping fitness divas DO give basic strength training a bad name.

The problem in fitness, however, is that because of this negative association with old-school training methods, the industry is going too far in the other direction. Anything even remotely basic in nature is considered worthless. Everything has to be new and cutting edge to be effective.

On a side note, is the cutting-edge stuff really effective? Many of the people I see balancing, flipping, bouncing, or meditating around don't look like they've ever stepped foot inside a gym.

Exercise fads come and go, but the basic exercises are the basics and have stood the test of time for a reason—because they work. This is a highly informed and intelligent way to train. And quite frankly, it's the most effective and efficient way to build and shape a body.

Sure, I may use some machines and isolated cable systems work for weak-point training and/or to correct muscle imbalances and computer posture, but the majority of the training should be focused on basic bodyweight, barbell, and dumbbell exercises (squat and deadlift variations, lunge variations, pull-ups, dips, push-ups, various free weight rows and presses, etc.).

If you can't get the job done with that, nothing more "cutting edge" is going to help you, despite the magic-pill marketing.

Build Muscle with Physique Parameters

The main benefits of isotonic exercise include improvements in muscular strength, power, hypertrophy, and endurance. Although you may see improvements in each of these categories for any given exercise, it is best to focus specifically on improving strength, power, hypertrophy, or endurance. You can accomplish this by adjusting the level of intensity or the number of sets and repetitions performed for each exercise, also known as the training load, to suit the desired area of improvement."—National Strength & Conditioning Association

So how do you train to build muscle? What does that look like on paper? What are the details and parameters of that type of program?

There is a principle in exercise physiology called the SAID principle: Specific Adaptation to Imposed Demands. All this really means is that your body adapts to the specific training that you do. It all comes down to adjusting the details of the program.

For the nerds, that means adjusting training frequency, volume, intensity, etc. Simply match the details of your training program to your training goals. If your goals change, your program should change.

Here's a chart that lays it all out for you (from the National Strength & Conditioning Association):

GOAL	FREQUENCY (per week)	LOAD & INTENSITY (% 1RM)	REPS	SETS	INTERSET REST
Strength	3-4	>85	<6	2-6	2-5 min
Power (single-effort)	1-2	80-90	1-2	3-5	2-5 min
Power (multiple-effort)	1-2	75-85	3-5	3-5	2-5 min
Hypertrophy	**3-5**	**60-85**	**6-20**	**3-6**	**30-90 seconds**
Endurance	5-7	<60	>20	2-3	<30 seconds

Traditional hypertrophy training is the fastest and most efficient way to change a body's physical appearance; this uses dumbbell and barbell exercises, multiple sets per exercise, moderate rep ranges, short-to-moderate interset rests, etc.

I know it's not new or flashy or innovative or cutting edge, but it damn sure is effective, and of all the possible adaptations to a training program, building muscle is the only thing that provides us with the most noticeable visual change, which is what we're after.

Given that I am in love with the mirror, if I thought any other mode of training was superior to this approach, I would be training my clients and myself in that method. I don't care about the program itself, I only care about the end result.

For example, if I thought cross-training or boot camp training was superior, I guarantee I'd be out there with my testicle-revealing soccer shorts and whistle. If I thought lightweight circuit training for the ladies was superior, I'd be working at Curves.

But alas, science, personal experience, and anecdotal evidence from some of the fittest-looking people in the world would concur with my opinion. Like Bruce Lee, I'm not tied to any dogmatic system. I just want what works—and traditional hypertrophy training works, no doubt about it.

Miyaki's Preferred Method: The Physique Cheat Sheet

The above charts are more for university students and professional trainers, and to be honest, are kind of incomplete. I have my own "cheat sheet" for building The Beach Physique. Here it is:

1. Train each muscle group once every 3-5 days. Beginners can do a full-body routine twice a week; Intermediates could do something like a 3-day alternating push/pull split (one week perform 2 push workouts and 1 pull workout, the next week perform 2 pull workouts and 1 push workout); and Advanced can do a 4-day upper body/lower body or 4-5-day body part split.
2. Perform 3-8 sets per muscle group per training session. That can be 1 exercise per muscle group for 3-8 sets (a la Vince Gironda or German Volume Training), or 2-3 sets of multiple exercises per muscle group (traditional bodybuilding).
3. Perform 8-20 reps per set, using 65-85% of your 1-rep max.
4. Use good form. To ensure good form, many trainers/coaches will recommend rep tempos. I like a 2-0-1-0 tempo: Lower the weight under control (two seconds)

and lift with some controlled force (one second). Don't pause or lockout your joints at either end of the motion (0 seconds at top/bottom).

5. Rest 30-90 seconds between each set.

Sample 3-Day Training Split

Workout A—Pull Day + Calves

Exercise	Sets	Reps	Interset Rest
Sumo Deadlift	3	8-12	90s
Close grip pull-ups or pulldowns	3	Maximum reps	90s
Chest supported dumbbell rows	3	8-12	60s
Barbell curls	3	8-12	60s
Dumbbell side lateral raises	3	12-15	45s
Cross-body hammer curls	3	12-15	45s
Calf raises	3	15-20	30s

Workout B—Push Day + Core

Exercise	Sets	Reps	Interset Rest
Split Squats or lunges	3	15-20 per side	90s
Flat dumbbell bench press	3	8-12	60s
Dips or push-ups	3	Maximum reps	60s
Incline dumbbell press	3	12-15	45s
Cable triceps extensions	3	12-15	45s
Hanging Leg Raises	3	Maximum reps	30s
Bicycle crunches	3	Maximum reps	30s

Step #6—Moderate Your Dietary Fat Intake

If you've been working your way down the checklist (like you should be——don't be skipping ahead Mr., Mrs., or Miss Impatient; the steps were organized this way due to their place in the hierarchy of importance)—you're now:

1. In a calorie deficit
2. Emphasizing predominantly high-satiety whole foods
3. Eating optimum levels of protein
4. Strength training a few times a week

Baby, those are the fundamental steps that are going to take you the majority of the way. The rest is just the details. If you are a beginner and need a little bit of a theoretical break, get out there and focus on practically applying those Fearsome Four steps first.

If you're ready to push forward with setting up your fully targeted fat-slashing plan, let's keep this thing rolling.

Flexibility with the Rest of Your Calories

We last left off our diet discussion with calorie deficits combined with optimum protein levels as the first two pieces of the puzzle. But we still have to fill in the rest of our calorie allotment with something.

For example, 150g of protein only equals 600 calories. Depending on your protein sources—lean to not-so-lean—that probably provides an additional 200-500 calories from the dietary fat within those protein foods (fish, meat, eggs, etc.). So we still have some extra energy nutrients (added carbs or fats) to eat.

Here's the unbiased truth: a variety of approaches can work for targeted fat loss once you control for a calorie deficit, optimal protein, good food choices, and consistent strength training. That's why you see so many heated debates at nutrition conferences and in fitness forums.

I don't get it. If you step back from the dogma and look at it from an objective perspective, real-world results prove a variety of approaches can work.

There are plenty of physique athletes who have gotten in great shape by following low-carb, higher-fat diets (again, within the confines of a calorie deficit). There are plenty of physique athletes who have gotten in great shape by following low-fat, higher-carb diets (within the confines of a calorie deficit). And there are plenty of physique athletes who have gotten into great shape by following a variety of approaches in between those two extremes, with more middle-of-the-road macronutrient ratios (within the confines of a calorie deficit).

Despite this variety of macronutrient approaches, what connects them is that they were all adhering to the steps higher up the hierarchy, whether they were aware of it or not (the most important being a calorie deficit).

Ultimately, it comes down to testing and assessing in the real world and finding out what macronutrient breakdown works best for you.

Now, that's not to say I can't give you my suggested starting points based on my own research and practical experience.

While I certainly believe a variety of macronutrient distributions can work, I believe that some are much better than others based on the principle of specificity (a geeky word that means appropriately matching the diet program to the training program and the person's individual needs and goals).

The diets that are the best for sedentary individuals just trying to improve their health and lose some weight are different than those of athletes and regular exercisers trying to reach elite shape and show off a 6-pack.

And I believe that some are better than others in terms of optimal energy, mood, immunity, natural hormone production, sexual function, ease and enjoyment of plan, and of course the most important, but most often overlooked, diet factor to consider—the long-term sustainability of a plan.

The Sedentary Person's Detour

Some research implies that lower-carb, Paleo-style diets may be the best approach for improving body composition and biomarkers of health for obese, insulin resistant, pre-diabetic, and sedentary populations.

It makes sense. If you don't burn a lot of carbs throughout the day, and your body has problems processing carbs, then cutting back on those carbs can be beneficial for both body fat reduction and improvements in biomarkers of health.

Personally, I have used such plans with corporate wellness programs and with deconditioned beginners to achieve some pretty amazing weight loss results.

What are the specifics of that approach? Well, of course, start at the top as always.

1. Get in the calorie deficit necessary for fat loss (10 cals/lbs of lean body mass or target bodyweight).
2. Set protein levels (0.7-1.0g/lbs of lean body mass or target bodyweight).
3. Then, limit carbs to roughly 100-125g a day, primarily coming from micronutrient dense, whole foods—an unlimited amount of non-starchy vegetables, 1-2 pieces of whole fruit, and 1 serving of starchy carbohydrates a day (rice or root vegetables).

4. Fill in the rest of your calories with healthy fats—fats as by-product of your high-quality animal protein sources and/or whole food fats like avocado and coconut.

To get this demographic started with an exercise routine, I emphasize mostly low-intensity activity (daily walking). Why? As you'll learn in the next chapter, I don't think low-carb diets combined with consistent, frequent, high-intensity anaerobic training are a great match.

First, the beginner and/or severely deconditioned individual needs to lose some weight and get healthier. The most efficient way to do this is to improve their diet and simply start the exercise habit with something that has a low barrier to entry (walking—you can do it anywhere, anytime, and it's not that challenging or taxing on the body).

Then they can think about increasing the intensity of their training for higher-level physique goals and add back in some frickin' carbs to support that anaerobic training.

I know that's not you because, after all, this is *The 6-Pack Checklist*. You, my advanced physique brother or sister, have been driven to insanity by vanity and are already strength training like a beast to build your beach physique.

But perhaps your coworker or your aunt's best friend could benefit by learning more about the details of this beginner's program. I wrote a whole book geared towards weight loss for beginners. It contains the step-by-step process I recommend for that specific demographic. Tell them they can check it out here: *The Truth about Weight Loss*

Or better yet, give it to them as a gift.

Carbs-Based Diets for Athletes & Regular Exercisers

To summarize, a relatively lower-carb diet that emphasizes protein, healthy fats, and whole foods as the foundation, along with some daily walking, is a great approach for the beginner, sedentary office worker, pre-diabetic, or severely deconditioned person trying to lose some weight and improve their health.

But you won't build a beach body and strut around with a sizzling 6-pack that way. To reach elite shape, you must hit the weights. You must earn your way to the upper echelon of fit physiques with high-intensity exercise.

We are going to talk a lot more about this in the next section, but high-intensity exercise changes everything when it comes to targeted diet design.

It creates a unique metabolic environment and an altered physiological state, and it changes the way your body processes nutrients for up to 48 hours after completion of a training session. If you exercise 3-5 days a week, then your body is virtually in a recovery mode 100% of the time. It is in an altered physiological state beyond pure resting conditions 100% of the time, thus its nutritional needs are completely different than that of the average sedentary office worker.

Since that's the case, I tend to lean more towards carb-based diets for those who perform high-intensity exercise on a regular basis—strength training, interval training, cross-training, intermittent sprint sports, tantric sex, etc. Here's why:

The body can't use fatty acids or ketones to fuel anaerobic metabolism. It must use glucose. That's geeky biochemistry, but it basically just means the body can't use fat to fuel your physique-focused strength-training sessions. It uses carbohydrates (or muscle glycogen that is made from carbohydrates).

Since that's the case, an adequate amount of carbs is necessary to help you properly fuel and recover from those physique-focused training sessions.

Why are we talking about this now in a section on dietary fats? Well, because the two are interrelated when it comes to designing a diet. More accurately, they should be inversely related. Why?

Remember, the overarching theme of our fat loss dream is that we need to be in a calorie deficit to slash fat and get lean. This fundamental principle impacts every other step of the diet design process.

Protein should remain relatively constant to support the maintenance of lean muscle mass. Carbs and fats are the only two macronutrients left. So if one goes up, the other must come down to consistently hit your fixed calorie deficit number. It's simple math.

When Carbs Go Up, Fats Should Come Down

> *Because carbs are not stored in the body, the optimal carb intake does not change when one is restricting calories. So dieters should continue to eat the same number of carbs . . . Similarly, protein intake should not change on a weight loss diet. Muscle is the body's primary storage reservoir for protein, and it is not desirable to lose muscle. So dieters should consume the same number of protein calories . . . Fat, however, is different. The body has a large internal store of fat, and any calorie deficit will be met by releasing fats from adipose tissue. So fat intake, strictly speaking, is not nutritionally necessary for an overweight person.*
> –Paul Jaminet

Changing your body composition comes down to varying your energy nutrient intake. We set our essential amino acid and essential fatty acid needs (primarily taken care of by animal protein, a good source of both) and never go below these base levels. Beyond that, all other food intake is just a source of energy.

We need to reduce our energy intake enough in order to create a deficit and force our bodies to tap into an internal reserve fuel source—body fat. We can do that by reducing carbohydrate intake, reducing fat intake, or both.

If you are an anaerobic athlete and/or perform strength training in order to build muscle and change your physique, cutting all carbs may not be the best approach, as they are the primary fuel for strength and speed sports. In this case, cutting down "added" dietary fats may be the more efficient path.

Given that we are leaning more towards carbohydrates to support strength-training sessions, dietary fat should be controlled.

I know we are living in a low-carb era. So for those who fear the carb during fat-slashing phases, just remember that total calories are still the most important step for fat loss. If you strength train while maintaining a relative calorie deficit, you can still include some starchy carbs in the diet while losing significant amounts of body fat.

The majority of the leanest people on Earth—natural bodybuilders and fitness models (yes, even the non-juiced up, non-crazy, non-OCD, perfectly healthy ones)—diet this way. Pre-contest diets include animal proteins, veggies, whole fruit, and some starch to support anaerobic training.

You shouldn't learn everything from gifted athletes because genetics and drugs often play a factor. But you can't completely ignore them either. The percentage of people who achieve success with the above approach is more than just coincidence. It is statistical significance. And success in the real world always leaves a few clues that the rest of us can use.

Here is one mistake, however, that I see happen time and time again in today's low-carb era. Someone is following a lower-carb/higher-fat/Paleo-style diet and combining it with consistent anaerobic training. They are suffering from some of the associated symptoms of this mismatched plan like poor performance, bad mood, anxiety or depression, muscle loss, stubborn fat, skinny-fat syndrome, insomnia, and lowered testosterone and/or thyroid production.

They decide to add some carbs back into their diet to better support the fueling and recovery demands of their training sessions. But they don't change anything else. Here is what they've missed. Adding carbs adds calories to their diet. So with the addition of carbs to their diet, they are now eating in a calorie surplus. What happens? They gain fat.

They falsely attribute this fat gain solely to the carbs (but it was actually because of an increase in total calories), condemn carbs as the starchy root of all evil, further increase their Nightmare on No-Carb Street, and go back to suffering through a mismatched diet.

Remember the hierarchy of importance and always start at the top of the 6-Pack Checklist.

You must keep calories the same if you want to truly test whether carbs are the bad guys or perhaps your best friends. Protein should stay constant to support lean muscle mass. That's why your carb and added fat intake must be inversely related. If you add carbs into your diet, you should remove an equal amount of dietary fat (and vice versa).

The Important Fat Factors

But you shouldn't cut dietary fat intake out completely as recommended in the low-fat era. Here are several reasons why.

1. We need a certain amount of essential fats to support normal functioning. These essential fats can't be made by the body and must be obtained through your diet.
2. We need a certain amount of fats as a transport medium for fat-soluble vitamins. How much?

    Consuming about 20g of dietary lipid daily provides a sufficient source to act as a transport medium for the fat-soluble vitamins A, D, E, and K.—McArdle, *Sports and Exercise Nutrition*

3. Certain fats have health benefits—increase HDL, lower LDL, improve insulin sensitivity, dilate blood vessels, lubricate joints, and support healthy hair and skin.
4. A certain amount of fat is necessary to support natural hormonal and enzymatic functioning—healthy fats support natural testosterone production, up-regulate fat-burning enzymes, etc.

Now, it's important to note here that there is an upper limit to how much increasing fats supports natural testosterone levels. People increasing dietary fat to say 70% of calories and thinking it is like taking steroids are sadly mistaken.

> *What can be concluded with current information is that very low-fat diets (<15-20 percent kcals from fat) can reduce testosterone, and consuming a moderate-fat diet will normalize testosterone. Furthermore, consuming a very high-fat diet (>40 percent calories from fat) compared to a moderate-fat (25-30 percent calories from fat) diet will not further increase testosterone.*
>
> –Layne Norton

From the article *"The Skinny on Dietary Fat and Testosterone."*

Keep Dietary Fat Moderate in Fat-Slashing Phases

How do we get the right amount of dietary fat to support normal functioning and natural hormone production, yet leave enough room for some carbs to fuel our strength-training sessions, all without inhibiting the fat loss process?

It's not as complicated as it sounds. The middle ground is where most of the magic lies for physique athletes.

1. Eat 0.20-0.33 g/lb of lean body mass or target bodyweight.

Miyaki's Preferred Method: Get Fat Predominantly as a By-Product of Your Protein Sources

What's the easiest way to hit those numbers?

1. Get the majority, if not all, of your dietary fat as a by-product of your animal protein sources (fish, meat, eggs) without "added" fats.

   Moderately lean animal proteins provide us with all of the essential fatty acids we need for normal functioning. These are much smaller than you think—just a few grams a day. It's almost impossible to become deficient in omega-6 fats, and a couple of servings of fish a week takes care of omega-3 fats.

   In other words, pounding butter, cream, and oils all day is not providing your body with essential nutrients. It's providing it with extra energy (aka calories). This can be good or bad depending on the situation.

Animal proteins also provide us with saturated fats, monounsaturated fats, and essential fats in the right amounts and ratios that Mother Nature intended. You can't beat nature.

2. If you happen to prefer really lean protein sources and need additional fats to meet your numbers, emphasize whole food fats (coconut, avocado, raw unsalted nuts).

    This will give you dietary fat in its highly satiating natural state—combined with protein and/or fiber—not in an altered/refined state that can easily lead to overconsumption, overshooting calorie levels, and gaining fat.

    Many of the bad characteristics of dietary fat for physique goals (just like many of the bad characteristics of carbohydrates)—including low food volume and low satiety—are a direct result of food refining.

3. I prefer cooking methods that do not use oil (grill; bake; broil; slow-cooker methods; stew in fish, chicken, or beef stocks; stir-fry with vegetables in its own juices, etc.).

4. If you cook with oil, stick to coconut, macadamia nut, or olive oil, and use as little as possible. More specifically, drizzle just enough for taste.

5. For condiments, choose lower calorie options—balsamic vinegar, soy sauce, salsa, mustard, fish sauce, soup stocks, salt and pepper, herbs and spices, boring and bland—so you are not adding a bunch of hidden calories to your base meals.

6. If you do use oil-based condiments like salad dressings, again, drizzle just enough for taste.

Step #7—Adjust Your Carbs as Necessary

Working our way down the checklist, here is where we currently stand:

1. We're in the calorie deficit necessary for fat loss.
2. We're cutting back on refined, processed, and hyperpalatable foods.
3. We're emphasizing predominantly high-satiety whole foods.
4. We're eating optimum levels of protein.
5. We're strength training a few times a week.
6. We are keeping our dietary fat intake moderate in order to leave some room for carbs.

From that point, the rest of the diet design is simple. In fact, it is so simple that there is no other choice—fill in all of your remaining calories with carbohydrates.

As I said in the last section, there are a variety of macronutrient breakdowns that can work for a targeted fat loss phase. But I've always believed the best ballpark starting point for the highest percentage of relatively healthy people trying to get ripped is this:

1. Keep carbs as high as possible to fuel and recover from anaerobic training while:
   - Eating enough protein to support lean muscle mass,
   - Eating a baseline level of fats to support normal functioning and natural hormone production, and
   - Staying in the calorie deficit necessary for optimum fat loss.
2. To accomplish the above:
   - Set calories at a level that is ideal for fat loss
   - Set protein and baseline fat intake
   - Fill in all remaining calories with carbohydrates
   - This will probably end up being in the range of 1-2g/lbs of lean body mass or target bodyweight

Now some may need to make adjustments from there and go lower in carbs to get lean. But if you are strength training or performing any other high-intensity activity on a regular basis, here are the many reasons why I suggest you give a carb-based approach a shot first, even if you are starting out with a lot of weight to lose.

The Case for Keeping Some Carbs in Your Fat-Slashing Diet

Since this book is about a checklist, practical strategies, and a step-by-step process, I don't want to bore the crap out of you before you get started with your plan. But I do think you should know a little bit about the "why" behind my recommendations, so you don't get caught up in the low-carb craze and end up with a mismatched diet approach that leads you down a dead-end road.

So let's summarize, list-style:

1. Those who only perform low-intensity aerobic activities can perform well on low-carb diets. However, low-carb diets negatively impact performance in higher intensity activities, like strength training and cross-training.

> *Carbohydrate availability may influence not only the performance of prolonged exercise but also the performance of intermittent-intensity and high-intensity exercise. Because carbohydrate is the most important fuel for the central nervous system, various cognitive tasks and motor skills that play a crucial role in skill sports may also be affected by carbohydrate availability.*
> –Asker Jeukendrup, Sports Nutrition

2. Chronic carb depletion combined with anaerobic training can eventually lead to muscle loss. The body will break down amino acids as a reserve fuel to provide the glucose necessary to fuel the brain and central nervous system at rest, as well as the muscles during high-intensity activity.

> *A low-carbohydrate diet rapidly depletes glycogen reserves, which severely affects one's ability to train hard and compete. This diet also sets the stage for loss of lean tissue as the body recruits amino acids from muscle to maintain blood glucose (gluconeogenesis)—an undesirable side effect for a diet designed for body fat loss . . . Protein use for energy reaches its highest level during exercise in a glycogen-depleted state*
> –Katch and McArdle, Sport and Exercise Nutrition

3. Carbs support optimum immune system functioning, especially given high-intensity training. Hard training can cause a temporary impairment of the immune system and increase susceptibility to illness. With consistent high-intensity exercise, adequate carb intake lessens the potentially negative changes in immunity brought about

by training. Many who combine low-carb diets with high-intensity training often complain of depressed immunity and getting sick all of the time.

> *Because elevated levels of stress hormones seem to cause many aspects of exercise-induced immune function impairment, nutritional strategies that effectively reduce the stress hormone response to exercise would be expected to limit the degree of exercise-induced immune dysfunction. The size of the glycogen stores in muscle and liver at the onset of exercise influence the hormonal and immune response to exercise . . . When people perform prolonged exercise following several days on very low-carbohydrate diets, the magnitude of the stress hormone (e.g., adrenaline and cortisol) and cytokine (e.g., IL-6, IL-1 ra, and IL-10) response is markedly higher than it is on normal-or high-carbohydrate diets . . . It has been speculated that athletes deficient in carbohydrate are placing themselves at risk from the immunosuppressive effects of cortisol and reduced glutamine availability, including the suppression of antibody production, lymphocyte proliferation, and NK cell cytotoxic activity."*
> –Asker Jeukendrup, Sports Nutrition

4. Sufficient carbohydrate intake supports an optimum free testosterone:cortisol ratio IN RESPONSE to high-intensity activity. Our industry focuses on how important dietary fat is for supporting natural testosterone levels in all populations, which it is, but carbohydrates also play a role specifically for athletes.

This study examined the effect of dietary carbohydrate (CHO) consumption on the free testosterone to cortisol (fTC) ratio during a short-term intense micro-cycle of exercise training. The fTC ratio decreased significantly from pre-study resting measurement to the final post-study resting measurement in the low-CHO group (-43%), but no change occurred in the control-CHO group (-3%). Findings suggest if the fTC ratio is utilized as a marker of training stress or imbalance it is necessary for a moderately high diet of CHO to be consumed to maintain validity of any observed changes in the ratio value.

Lane et al. **Influence of dietary carbohydrate intake on the free testosterone: cortisol ratio responses to short-term intensive exercise training.** <u>Eur J Appl Physiol.</u> 2010 Apr;108(6):1125-31.

5. Low-carb diets coupled with intense training protocols can impair thyroid production and sabotage normal metabolic rate. More specifically, it can impair the conversion of T4 thyroid hormone to its more active T3 form. This can impair fat loss and cause a chronic state of fatigue and sluggishness.

6. A carb-depleted state can affect the natural production of neurotransmitters like serotonin and dopamine. This can cause insomnia, depression, anxiety, and irritability.

Moderate Carb Diets for Physique & Fat Loss

Most sports nutrition diets assume the goal is to maximize glycogen stores in between training sessions in order to optimize performance. As a result, they tend to be on the high side of carbohydrate recommendations.

Recommendations developed on behalf of the International Olympic Committee by experts in Sports Nutrition. Carbohydrate recommendations 5-7 g/kg bw during regular training needs and 7-10g/kg bw during periods of increased training. The recovery period should be no less than 24 hours (for glycogen restoration).–Burke et al.

But it is important to keep in mind that the needs and goals of PERFORMANCE athletes are different than that of a PHYSIQUE enthusiast.

The training of performance-based athletes tends to be higher in duration and frequency—they may train 2-4 hours a day, sometimes twice a day. This is unnecessary for physique development. A traditional hypertrophy routine consists of 3-4, 40-60 minute strength-training workouts a week. So performance athletes generally have much higher calorie and carbohydrate demands.

In addition, achieving high levels of performance is much different than achieving low levels of body fat. A little body fat is acceptable to the performance athlete as long they are performing at optimal levels. In fact, getting too low in body fat at some point hinders performance.

Body fat is not acceptable to the physique athlete. The physique athlete is willing to sacrifice some performance output in order to attain the lowest levels of body fat and the maximum leanness.

Ten grams of carbohydrate per kg of bodyweight for a 165lb male would equal 750g of carbohydrate per day. While you might have a ton of energy and perform well with that number, I would argue that most would have a very hard time getting lean.

The physique enthusiast needs to find the middle ground between the lower carbohydrate recommendations for the sedentary and the very high carbohydrate recommendations for performance athletes.

The goal is to provide just enough carbohydrates to properly fuel and recover from strength-training sessions without any excess being stored as body fat.

This generally falls somewhere in the range of 1-2g/lb of lean body mass or target bodyweight, all within the confines of a calorie deficit.

Carb Quotes and Notes

Carbs are the most highly controversial and hotly debated topic in the diet, fitness, and fat loss industries today. You now know where I stand. But I would never ask you to just take my word for it.

> *It is good to consult with someone of good sense. An advisor will fulfill the way when he makes a decision by selfless and frank intelligence because he is not personally involved. This way of doing things will certainly be seen by others as being strongly rooted. It is, for example, like a large tree with many roots. One man's intelligence is like a tree that has been simply stuck in the ground.*
> —Hagakure

Here's what some of the best physique coaches I know of have to say on the topic:

> *For a bodybuilder, though, carbs have a more important role in energy for workouts, protein (muscle) sparing, and to stimulate metabolism than for the average person. In my opinion, especially during contest dieting, this makes dropping fat intake to 15-20% of overall calories beneficial as it makes more room for carbs and protein. For a sedentary or moderately training individual, lesser protein requirements and a more flexible diet plan can allow for a higher percentage of dietary fat . . . Carbs are the most protein-sparing nutrient we eat. If carbs are too low for too long, you'll lose muscle no matter how much protein you eat, period!*
> –Dr. Joe Klemczewski, from *The Truth About Fat and Getting Lean*

> *In a study of athletes taking in the same amount of protein (1.6 g/kg) during weight loss, performance decrements and LBM losses were avoided when adequate carbohydrate was maintained and dietary fat was lowered [13]. Mettler, et al. [29] also found that a caloric reduction coming from dietary fat while maintaining adequate carbohydrate intake and increasing protein to 2.3 g/kg maintained performance and almost completely eliminated LBM losses in resistance trained subjects.*
> –Eric Helms

Helms et al. **Evidence-based recommendations for natural bodybuilding contest preparation: nutrition and supplementation.** Journal of the International Society of Sports Nutrition 2014, 11:20 doi:10.1186/1550-2783-11-20.

The no-carb crew believes that fat can only be burned when carbs are kept close to zero or under 50 grams a day—about that found in a small apple and a single thin slice of bread. That's not true. As long as you eat fewer carbs along with fewer calories than you typically eat on a daily basis, you will start to burn some body fat. Plus extreme low-carb dieting poses a few problems. Near carb-free diets completely zap your energy levels, which downgrades the metabolic rate. In a rush to lose fat fast, the individual who slashes carbs across the board will often create a downdraft in the metabolic rate—the total calories burned each day. So while he begins to eat radically less calories and carbs, the body often compensates by downgrading its metabolism.

The other negative; those who train with weights using a very low-carb diet often lose muscle because you need an adequate carbohydrate intake to preserve and hold muscle mass. When carbs are cut too low, you burn a lot of muscle while you train. When you burn muscle, you initiate a drop in metabolism because the total amount of muscle one carries is directly linked to burning calories. When you have a lot of muscle, you burn a lot of calories and when you add muscle, you upgrade your metabolism. On the other hand, when you burn muscle, you downgrade your metabolism. I call it dumb dieting. Most dieters who train with weights can see great results by modifying their carb intake from 2 or more grams recommended in the mass gaining phase to 1 to 1.5 grams per pound of bodyweight in order to cut up. That would mean a 200 pound bodybuilder or athlete eating 400 or more grams daily to build mass would drop down to 200 to 300 grams to cut up—without resorting to extreme low carbs, which has the potential to cause a quick drop in muscle mass and metabolism.

–Chris Aceto, author of Championship Bodybuilding

Miyaki's Preferred Method: A Moderate Carb Approach for Physique Transformation

To summarize this annoyingly long section and my preferred fat loss diet starting point in general:

1. Set calories at 11-13 cals/lb of lean body mass or target bodyweight.
2. Set protein at 0.7-0.9g/lb of lean body mass or target bodyweight, rounding up to 1.0g/lb if you wish.
3. Set dietary fat at 0.2-0.33g/lb of lean body mass or target bodyweight. The majority should come as a by-product of your protein sources.
4. Fill in all remaining calories with carbohydrates. This will likely fall in the range of 1-2g/lb of lean body mass or target bodyweight.

If you'd like to learn more about the details, science, and strategies regarding targeted carbohydrate intake and fat loss diet numbers in general, you can check out my book *The Truth about Carbs*.

Step #8—Ditch the Fitness Myths & Find a Sustainable Diet Structure

The details of our diet plan are all set—an average calorie deficit, targeted macronutrients, and good food choices.

Now it is time to transition to a bigger picture issue—diet structure. Although this step is lower down the hierarchy of importance when it comes to the pure physiological aspects of a fat loss diet (and getting a 6-pack), it is perhaps number one in terms of importance when it comes to diet practicality, sustainability, and thus, long-term adherence rates.

It doesn't matter if you have the greatest plan in the world written down on a piece of paper. If you can't make that plan work in the real world and actually stick to it on a consistent basis, it is meaningless.

Regardless of what diet you follow and its recommended diet numbers or food templates, it seems that the assumed diet-structure standard is the fitness nutrition, six-gun spread. Take whatever you are supposed to eat and spread it out over six small meals or snacks every few hours.

Most plans also recommend tapering your calorie and food intake over the course of the day—eat earlier in the day, and then cut calories and try to starve on protein shakes and lettuce leaves at night.

Geez. Lugging around Tupperware to your meetings, watching the clock, having your life revolve around your diet, and trying to fall asleep thinking about gnawing off your significant other's arm. That sounds fun, huh?

A Sane Diet Structure is the Key to Sustainability

Fitness nutrition recommendations work, and they work quite well. Many natural bodybuilders, fitness models, and other fitness professionals get in tremendous shape following this structure.

I have used such plans in the past myself and achieved great results. I have worked with both performance and physique athletes who have done the same. It certainly is a viable option if that structure fits into your lifestyle. So I'm not one of these dudes dissing proven methods and saying alternative methods are the only answer.

But it's just that I've also worked with real people in the real world for over fifteen years, and what I've discovered is that for 90% of us with careers, families, social lives, and sex lives, the traditional fitness nutrition approach is impractical and unsustainable for the long term.

Why do you think we have so many fitness magazines and diet books coming out every month but so few people actually making any fat loss progress? These programs are nice to read about for entertainment purposes and when envisioning the ideal situation in theory, but they are hard to execute in the real game-time situations of everyday life.

Hitting a punching bag is one thing. Hitting a moving target that is also swinging back (real life with new challenges and obstacles popping up every day) is something completely different.

The key question is this: Is the traditional fitness diet structure absolutely necessary to get optimal physique transformation results? Or are there some alternative methods that give relatively sane people a better shot at succeeding?

Unbiased Science vs. Engrained Tradition

Here's the truth. Numerous scientific studies have shown that if you eat the same calories and foods, meal frequency is irrelevant in terms of fat loss.

Meal Frequency and Energy Balance

Although some short-term studies suggest that the thermic effect of feeding is higher when an isoenergetic test load is divided into multiple small meals, other studies refute this, and most are neutral. More importantly, studies using whole-body calorimetry and doubly-labelled water to assess total 24 h energy expenditure find no difference between nibbling and gorging. There is no evidence that weight loss on hypoenergetic regimens is altered by meal frequency. We conclude that any effects of meal pattern on the regulation of body weight are likely to be mediated through effects on the food intake side of the energy balance equation.—British Journal of Nutrition

That's really just a fancy/geeky way of saying that despite what you've heard in the fitness industry, you can get equally good fat loss results eating 6, 3, or even 2 main meals a day.

Since that's the case, you can build your diet plan around your lifestyle, natural tendencies, career demands, daily schedule, time and food availability, etc. You can make the diet fit your life as opposed to the other way around.

The optimum meal frequency pattern—FOR YOU—is the one that allows you to be the most consistent with your diet. Whatever pattern is the most practical, functional, sustainable, and effective for you, given your specific situation and goals, is the best pattern for YOU. Don't cling to archaic traditions or modern gurus.

To slave away trying to fit into a fitness approach of six small meals a day may be unrealistic and counterproductive, and, most important, it's completely unnecessary. Once people let go of this myth, most do a lot better with adherence, and thus success rates, by reducing their meal frequency to more normal and doable patterns.

You might try out, I don't know, something like breakfast, lunch, and dinner . . .

The Truth About the Traditional Three Meals a Day Pattern

The three square meals a day approach gets bashed in the health and fitness industry and is often criticized as being counterproductive for weight loss.

However, this is most likely due to the fact that the typical Y2K Diet is used as the representative of this approach—mocha and pastry for breakfast, sandwich and chips for lunch, pizza and ice cream for dinner. It looks a lot like "the Cafeteria Diet" from the study we mentioned in a previous chapter.

This is problematic for comparison because these are not the typical meals eaten by someone pursuing weight loss or body composition transformation. The suboptimal food choices are the problem, not the meal frequency pattern itself.

Three meals a day can work great for weight loss provided you are making good food choices.

To contrast, the traditional Japanese diet yields some of the lowest obesity and diabetes rates in the world. A three-meal pattern for that would look something like this: eggs and rice for breakfast; chicken, veggies, and rice for lunch; fish, veggies, and rice for dinner.

Maybe you are starting to see why I believe there is a hierarchy of importance when it comes to fat loss. If crappy food choices are causing you to consistently eat in caloric excess, no diet structure is going to help you slash fat and get lean. I don't give a damn if you are eating 24 meals a day, on the hour, every hour.

Conversely, if good food choices are helping you stay in the average caloric deficit necessary for fat loss, virtually any meal frequency and food distribution pattern can work well.

Three for Sustainability

So assuming you are properly working your way down the 6-Pack Checklist, both fitness nutrition spreads and the traditional three-meals-a-day pattern can work equally well. The difference?

The traditional three is a lot more practical for about 80% of the non-fitness professional population. Maybe you should give it a shot.

And, in fact, research shows three protein-based meals a day is a great strategy for losing weight and maintaining high levels of satiety along the way. We mentioned the following study in the section on optimizing protein intake, but as a courtesy to you so you don't have to flip back through, I'm repeating it here:

Eating fewer, regular-sized meals with higher amounts of lean protein can make one feel more full than eating smaller, more frequent meals, according to new research from Purdue University. We found that when eating high amounts of protein, men who were trying to lose weight felt fuller throughout the day; they also experienced a reduction in late-night desire to eat and had fewer thoughts of food.

We also found that despite the common trend of eating smaller, more frequent meals, eating frequency had relatively no beneficial impact on appetite control. The larger meals led to reductions in appetite, and people felt full. We want to emphasize though that these three larger meals were restricted in calories and reflected appropriate portion sizes to be effective in weight loss. Our advice for people trying to lose weight is to add a moderate amount of protein at three regular meals a day to help appetite control and the feeling of fullness.

Leidy HJ et al. **Influence of higher protein intake and greater eating frequency on appetite control in overweight and obese men.** Obesity (Silver Spring). 2010 Mar 25.

Stop Trying to Starve at Night

I've had a lot of breakthrough moments in my career, times where new research and experiences led to new strategies that I could apply to my diet and then teach to others. The goal has always been trying to get more consistent and sustainable fat loss results.

There has been one strategy that has positively impacted both my own and my clients' physique results more than all of the rest—combined! That's why it has become the key, core principle of my dietary approach.

Feast at night. That's right. Regardless of whatever meal frequency pattern you choose (the traditional three, more fitness-style small meal spreads, intermittent fasting, etc.), save a significant percentage of your calorie and carb intake so you can have a complete, satiating dinner at night. Escalate carb and calorie intake up throughout the day vs. tapering it down.

I know that goes against everything you normally hear in the fitness industry, but if everything you heard in the fitness industry actually worked, there'd be a lot more people walking around in great shape.

Flipping the script and eating big at night is the one step you can take today that will make your diet plan infinitely easier and more enjoyable to follow.

It is the one step that has helped my busy professional clients finally get great results, even those who had failed on multiple diet plans in the past and had all but given up.

As I'm writing this, I realize how much that sounds like infomercial BS, but it's The Truth, and I think you can handle it. I truly believe it will help you and that once you try it, you'll never go back to any other way of eating again. Here are several reasons why I believe it works so well:

1. Evolutionary Instinct

Human beings evolved on a fasting and feeding cycle. We spent the majority of our existence eating lighter during the day while actively tracking, hunting, and gathering our food. We spent the evening relaxing and feasting on the majority, if not all, of our daily food intake.

So it's our natural instinct to eat big at night, based on thousands of years of evolution. For some odd and inexplicable reason, most diet plans work off a structure that goes completely against this (eat big during the day and then try to cut calories and carbs, and starve at night). That's why most diet plans suck in terms of long-term adherence.

To give yourself the best shot at succeeding beyond a 60-day time frame, or whatever, I believe you should go with, not against, your nature.

2. Natural Social Patterns

Socially, most of us want to eat big at night. Think about it—enjoying a meal with your family at night, going out with friends or on a date, doing business over dinner, etc.

No one wants to starve on lettuce leaves and be preoccupied with how much their diet sucks when they could be eating a satiating meal like a steak and potato and getting equally good weight loss and physique results.

3. Diet Psychology

Our brains work on a sacrifice-reward pattern. Most people find it relatively easy to cut calories, eat lighter, and make better food choices during the day, as long as they know they can eat a larger meal at night and get to end the day satiated and satisfied (at least in the kitchen; the bedroom is your own responsibility).

This is way more effective than large lunches that lead to rebound hypoglycemia and energy crashes, and tiny dinners that lead to starvation-induced, junk food binges.

Ditching Fitness Nutrition Myths

Eat the social norm of three meals a day and fulfill your natural desire to feast at night. Live like a normal person but look like a fitness model. It sounds awesome and like a sustainable lifestyle plan to you, rather than a miserable fitness diet you suffer through.

But alas, you have a few burning questions due to lingering fitness myths. That burning sensation? Baby, you might want to get that checked out. But as for the questions . . .

"Don't I have to eat small meals to rev up my metabolism or keep my muscles from falling off their bones?" "Won't eating a big meal with carbs at night cause me to store fat?"

Eating at night doesn't make you fat. Eating too much over the course of an entire day makes you fat. If you've eaten large and/or frequent meals throughout the day and then eat another large dinner on top of that, chances are you will overshoot your daily calorie needs and gain fat. It's the total food intake—not the distribution—that is the problem.

If you eat lighter during the day and are active, chances are you enter dinner in a relatively large calorie deficit with depleted energy reserves. Even a large meal with a significant amount of carbohydrates will be used to restore energy reserves first before spilling over into fat stores.

Even simpler, if you drive your car around all day and the gas tank is empty, you can and should fill up for the next day.

When we look at evolutionary history, it is clear that for most of our existence, we ate the biggest meal with the majority of our calories at night. I suggest we do the same if we want to make our diet plans as easy AND effective as possible.

Yet with fitness tradition, the advice to eat big at night seems controversial or counterintuitive. Almost every mainstream diet plan and fitness article recommends the opposite. At this point, we can use some research to clarify, or at least give you the courage to try something different to see if it works for you.

What do you have to lose? If you are reading this book, chances are whatever you are doing right now isn't working. Whatever you have tried in the past didn't work. Or it worked to achieve a short-term goal, but you are looking for a more sustainable style. Why not give something else a shot?

Here is a study supporting the theory that eating a higher percentage of your calories and carbs at night can work just as well, if not better, for targeted fat loss.

This study was designed to investigate the effect of a low-calorie diet with carbohydrates eaten mostly at dinner on anthropometric, hunger/satiety, biochemical, and inflammatory parameters . . . Greater weight loss, abdominal circumference, and body fat mass reductions were observed in the experimental diet in comparison to controls.

Sofer et al. 2011. **Greater weight loss and hormonal changes after 6 months diet with carbohydrates eaten mostly at dinner.** *Obesity (Silver Spring)* Oct;19(10):2006-14.

Some Potential Diet Structure Options

To review, the main principle of my recommended diet structure is to eat a larger percentage of your calories and carbs at night.

From there, based on personal experience and conversations with colleagues, I have come to believe there is a Bell Curve distribution of meal frequency patterns that end up being the most effective, practical, functional, and sustainable for people living in today's material world.

Fitness Nutrition Spreads—For 10-20% of the population, 5-6 small meals/snacks a day works great.

The Traditional Three—For 60-80% of the population or so (and the majority of busy professionals), the most functional approach seems to be to base your diet on three protein-based meals a day. After all, this is the pattern that society and civilization has set up as the normal structure in most cultures.

Intermittent Fasting—For the remaining 10-20% of the population, eating fewer than three meals a day may be the easiest plan to follow.

There is a series of dietary approaches collectively referred to as intermittent fasting. The overall philosophy involves reducing meal frequency; going through longer periods without food (fasting) to prolong the amount of time the body is in an energy producing, detoxifying, and fat-burning mode; and narrowing down the window of time within which you eat larger meals (feeding window) to ensure full nutritional replenishment and lean muscle mass maintenance.

A popular version of this approach is to fast for 16 hours and eat all of your daily food intake in an 8-hour window. In simpler terms, skip breakfast and eat all of your food for the day at lunch and dinner. This was popularized by Martin Berkhan of Leangains, and is also recommended by Paul Jaminet and his *Perfect Health Diet*.

Another version is to fast all day, or alternatively eat lighter, low-glycemic foods like fruits, vegetables, and small servings of protein during the day, and eat one main meal at night. This was popularized by Ori Hofmekler and his *Warrior Diet*.

But I want to reiterate that I called my approach intermittent feasting for a reason, to distinguish it from intermittent fasting. My main piece of advice, mostly from a practicality standpoint, is to "save" a significant portion of your calories and carbs for a satiating meal at night. What you do during the day to do that is flexible. Intermittent fasting is one of several options, but it is not a mandatory operating principle in my approach.

You might be thinking to yourself, "Great, Miyaki, do whatever I want. I get it. But what is your preferred style and suggested starting point from which I can go out and test, assess, and refine?"

Miyaki's Preferred Method: The 3 & Feast Strategy

Eat 3 protein-based meals a day—the traditional breakfast, lunch, and dinner.

Escalate your carb intake, and eat the highest percentage of your calories and carbs at night.

Keep your daytime meals to a carb:pro ratio of 1:1 or less.

Sample 3 & Feast Template:
Breakfast

- 1 serving of animal protein (3 eggs or leftover meat, fish, poultry, etc.)
- 1 piece of whole fruit

Lunch

- 1-2 servings of animal protein (meat, fish, poultry, etc.)
- 1 serving of starchy carbohydrates (rice or root vegetables)
- Optional: any non-starchy vegetables

Dinner

- 1-3 servings of animal protein (meat, fish, poultry, etc.)
- 1-4 servings of starchy carbohydrates (rice or root vegetables)
- Optional: any non-starchy vegetables

- ♦ Adjust your serving sizes based on your specific calorie and macronutrient numbers.
- ♦ 1 serving of animal protein = about the size of a deck of cards or iPhone
- ♦ 1 serving of starch = about the size of a baseball or closed fist

Miyaki's Alternative Methods

Remember, my style is just a suggested starting point. You have the flexibility and freedom to test, assess, refine, and ultimately find what works best for you. That last tidbit often gets lost.

Is intermittent fasting an option? Absolutely. If you want to go that route, all you would do is skip the breakfast and place those foods later in the day as a bigger lunch or dinner or a mid-afternoon snack.

And contrary to getting pigeonholed into a specific style, I've never abandoned fitness nutrition spreads as an option either. If you want to go that route, you could take some of the food from lunch and dinner and spread it out more evenly.

Although, again, for ease of plan, I would still save at least a decent portion of your calories and carbs for dinner.

Step #9—Add NEPA if Necessary

Remember the big picture view of our physique transformation approach:

1. We're using diet for 80% of our fat loss results.
2. In order to ensure the effectiveness of that approach, we are consistently adhering to the details of that diet—getting into a calorie deficit, emphasizing high-quality foods, hitting targeted macronutrient numbers, and using a practical diet structure that suits our style.
3. We're strength training a few times a week to build lean muscle mass and to shape, tighten, and tone the body.

In my opinion, that is a highly effective, efficient, and sustainable approach to slashing fat and living lean year-round, without having to give up your career, sanity, or social life. But I don't know. I could very well be a crazy fitness person who doesn't know he's crazy . . .

Regardless, let's call the above fundamental 6-pack principles our baseline, year-round, decently lean physique routine.

But what should you do if those steps fail to take you all the way to your physique goals? What if you hit a plateau in your initial fat loss efforts on the way down to your new, lower body fat set point? What if you have some stubborn fat that is hanging on for dear life? What other steps can you take to turn things up and get ultra-ripped for a specific event (photo shoot, competition, wedding, reunion, summer vacation, etc.)?

First, why so many frickin' questions? I ask one in return. What are you, the Riddler?

Second, that's what the last couple of steps down the checklist are all about. We'll call them the 6-Pack Troubleshooting Steps.

My first play call in that championship physique game situation is a little increase in NEPA.

NEPA Know How

If diet takes care of 80% of your fat loss, and you are already strength training to build/maintain your lean muscle mass, what else can you add to your plan to reach your physique peak and the final 20% of your fat loss goals?

Increase your informal, non-exercise-specific physical activity (NEPA).

In real-world terms, walk more as part of your day. Go for a walk in the morning, before lunch to take care of an errand, or before dinner with your kids. Go for a hike on the weekend.

Another fun (and truly functional) example of an increase in NEPA is to spend a little more "sexy time" with your significant other . . .

Caveman vs. Computer Dude

What's wrong with modern society? We just sit around too much. Human beings were made to move. We can always look back through evolutionary history to see what we should be doing for optimum health sans the modern obesity epidemic.

For most of our existence, we were hunters and gatherers. For most of the day, we performed sub-maximal activities. We walked around, gathered food, tracked prey, cooked, cleaned, etc. We may have sprinted towards prey or away from predators (anaerobic activity, like adding interval cardio or strength training), but 90% of our activity came in the form of walking.

We didn't run to keep the heart rate up or "hit some cardio." And we certainly didn't ride a stationary bike, pedal away on an elliptical, run on a treadmill to exercise for the sake of exercising, or try to formally "burn off" calories to make up for last night's ice cream bender.

None of what we did was formal exercise; we just completed the necessary tasks of the day, whatever that might have been. In fact, we used as little energy as possible during most of the day in order to conserve energy for when it was absolutely necessary for survival.

And when it was time to move, we frickin' moved, baby. We sprinted away from predators or towards prey. We climbed trees, hoisted objects, swung weapons, and clubbed stuff to death with maximal exertion. These are all predominantly anaerobic activities.

We're not meant to reach arbitrary fat-burning zones for arbitrary amounts of time. We're meant to alternate periods of kicking back with periods of kicking ass. That's how you efficiently build a functional, lean physique.

Take a Hike, Pal

> *High-Intensity Interval Training (HIIT) has become a conditioning staple. But what about another simple but hugely effective fat-stripping activity, namely steady-state walking? Fact is, for the typical reader that's muscular, lifts weights regularly, and might want to get a bit more cut, walking can be the perfect complement to a rigorous weight lifting routine . . .*
> *However, if on a diet and lifting weights, glycogen stores are depleted. If you add regular intense cardio on top of this, the body will release cortisol to help convert amino acids into glucose to be used as fuel. Those amino acids can come from your hard-earned muscle tissue . . . Fancy energy system workouts and complex lactic acid routines are fun and definitely effective, but they aren't mandatory if you want to get into great condition. The fact is, to get lean, you needn't look further than your own two legs. Walk, lift, and follow a reasonable diet, and the leanness will come.*
> –Tim Henriques from *Get Ripped. Get Walking*

Most people underestimate the power of simply attempting to walk more during a typical day. Yet a few of the most successful natural bodybuilders of all-time—John Hansen and Dave Goodin—shun traditional cardio in favor of outdoor walking in their pre-contest routines.

They know that walking is a small yet powerful tool in their fitness arsenal. Here are some of the specific benefits:

1. Walking can give us many of the same benefits as traditional cardio—calorie burn, increased cardiovascular efficiency, lowered blood pressure, etc.—without all of the drawbacks—joint wear and tear, repetitive strain, negative hormonal impact (overdoing traditional cardio can lead to increased cortisol output and testosterone suppression).

   It increases blood flow with minimal stress on the nervous, hormonal, and muscular systems. This may actually help you recover from intense strength-training sessions, whereas most other forms of cardio training would impair that recovery process.

2. It is convenient. It can be done anytime, anywhere, and can be squeezed in to any part of the day (even multiple times), not as a "formal" training session you have to plan for. No equipment, change of clothes, or commute to the gym is necessary.

3. It is not as boring as staring at a wall. With some outdoor walking, you get varied stimulus—buildings, trees, restaurants, blue sky, hot girls or guys (whatever you prefer) out on the town, etc., all depending on where you decide to go.

4. It is a good stress reliever. With the high stress of corporate jobs and modern living, walking is a good way to unwind, take your mind off things, and let your brain relax. If work is stressing you out, you are anxious and tense, and you feel like you are going to kill your boss or yourself, take a walk to clear your head. It helps.

   Listen, I'm too much of a stubborn, meathead athlete (I am not sitting or lying around for extended periods of time), a workaholic (that's where my mind goes these days when there's free time), and a pervert (I think you know what I'm saying with this one) to meditate. It just doesn't work for me.

But somehow, when I'm walking, I'm able to clear my mind and relax a little bit. It is kind of like my active meditation—my body needs to be moving for the cartoon I have going on up in my head to turn off for half an hour. Maybe it will work for you, too?

5. Because it is a leisurely activity, you can multi-task. You can take a walk with a friend or family member to catch up. That's probably better for your health and physique goals than catching up over a mocha and scone.

You can "talk business" or have an informal meeting with a colleague or client while walking somewhere. That's probably better than sitting right in front of them in an enclosed office wanting to rip their head off.

It's an active way to spend some time with your kids—they love to just go out and explore.

You can even be annoying cell phone guy or girl while walking.

Miyaki's Preferred Method: Off-Day Walks

1. Start with taking a 30-60 minute walk on your off days from strength training.
2. If you really need to ramp things up, take a daily walk.

Step #10—Track Your Food Intake if You're Having Trouble

As I have stated from the start of this book, consistently hitting the right numbers is the most important step to achieving any higher-level physique goal, including shredding down to a sizzling 6-pack.

You could be doing everything else right—making good food choices, never skipping your strength-training sessions, walking on a daily basis—but if you're overshooting your target diet numbers either because of your portion sizes, or more likely because extra hidden calories are sneaking into your days, you won't lose body fat.

When clients ask, "Why have I hit a plateau?" or "Why can't I lose that last layer, that last 5-10lbs?" I usually dig into the numbers to find the answer. As the great Brian Fantana once said, "60% of the time, it works all the time."

Actually, in my experience, it's been 95% of the time. How do you make sure you don't fall victim to the sneaky Calorie Creeper? I suggest you track your food intake and diet numbers.

"That's a pain in the butt." "I'm not a fitness freak." "I have a life."

Yeah, I know, but this is not something I recommend you do indefinitely. I don't track my food intake anymore. I gravitate towards certain foods and can now eyeball portion sizes like a hawk. But I highly suggest it at two different points in your fitness journey:

1. When you are first starting out.
2. When you want to ramp things up, reach higher-level physique goals, or peak for a certain event (a reunion, a wedding, for photos, for a summer vacation).

Here is why.

Education, Awareness, & Focus

Tracking shows you how the typical foods and meals you eat impact your diet numbers, which in turn impacts your ability to lose fat.

Are you "eating healthy" or "eating low-fat" or "eating Paleo" or "eating low-carb" but still not losing weight? Unless you are a genetic anomaly, you won't lose weight in a calorie surplus no matter how cutting edge or "metabolically advantaged" your diet plan supposedly is.

What do your macronutrient numbers look like? Maybe you are going too low in carbs and too high in fats, and workouts and recovery are suffering? We can feel like we are doing things right, but objective numbers tell the true story. Or, fat loss numbers never lie.

By simply tracking food intake and numbers for a week, I've had clients realize their protein intake was paltry, they were committing "carbicide" like Bruno, or they were eating 1000 calories per day above maintenance levels via refined oils. In short, they were not eating nearly as "good" as they thought they were.

By getting on track(ing tools), you'll get to know what your general serving sizes should be in order to hit your optimal fat loss numbers. You'll also probably see how much extra stuff is sneaking in there.

After you cut the excess crap and get a good feel for the right portions for you, then you can start to eyeball everything. You don't have to be a statistician forever, but it definitely helps educate and guide you in the beginning.

It is no different than tracking your spending habits or expenses when you are having trouble with your personal finances or business cash flow. You have to get to know where your money is coming in from and where it is leaking out—too many "business" lunches at adult entertainment establishments, huh?

That means you, ladies——I know your "Thunder From Down Under" secrets.

Flexibility & Sustainability

As you know from earlier in the book, I recommend an island-style diet. I believe you should stick to that the majority of the time for overall health, digestive health, and the satiety impacts of food.

But the unbiased truth is you can reach your physique goals as long as you hit your diet numbers, regardless of what foods you eat.

What if you shoot for good food choices 80-90% of the time to balance the ideal with the practical and sustainable? With tracking, you can still hit your numbers despite a little more leeway with your food choices.

Despite tracking being a little bit of a pain in the butt in the short-term, it creates a lot more dietary flexibility in the long-term. Want to work in some different foods to your "living lean year-round" lifestyle plan? Don't want to give up bread and pasta forever? Dig the occasional dessert?

Cool, just make sure your occasional food choices off the template fit within your targeted diet numbers for the day, and you'll keep slashing that fat away.

You'll also see how any meal at any restaurant can fit into your target numbers for the day. No more "I have to eat out all of the time" excuses.

You can eat for fat loss anywhere if you hit your numbers. This is key for an uptown girl, a downtown professional, or anyone else who eats the majority of their meals away from home.

Informed Adjustments to Bust Through Plateaus

Going from out of shape to decent shape is one thing. But going from good shape to the cover of a fitness magazine is a whole other thing. If you want to jump to the next physique class, this often necessitates being more detailed and consistent with your diet numbers.

I should rephrase that to be more accurate. It's not often. It is every time.

Busting through plateaus does not always necessitate biohacks or cutting edge strategies. Sometimes it actually necessitates the opposite—getting back to the boring basics.

The more ambitious your goals become, the more detailed and disciplined you need to be to achieve them. It is no different than any other profession or venture. For example, getting out of debt is one thing. Getting rich is another.

High-level physique goals are really fitness's closest version to high-level athletic goals. They require a little more sacrifice, discipline, and effort than that of a general health and fitness enthusiast.

You wouldn't just jump out of your office chair today and expect to win the Super Bowl or Ironman Triathlon tomorrow, simply by winging it, just because you suddenly wanted to. Yet that's the mistaken mentality many have when it comes to shedding fat and chasing 6-packs.

So if you are struggling to reach your high-level 6-pack goal and are only hitting your target diet numbers 80% of the time, you need to bump that average up to 90%.

If all has been on point on a consistent basis, maybe it's time to reassess and adjust the numbers for continued progress. But that step should only be taken if you've actually been sticking to your current numbers for a consistent period of time.

Otherwise, you're just changing stuff for the sake of it without ever having given it a chance to work. Nothing could be more meaningless.

See what I'm saying?

Miyaki's Preferred Method: The Tracking Tool Options

These days, with food databases and even smartphone apps, it's relatively easy to track your numbers. Here are a few free resources I recommend:

OPTION #1—PEN & PAPER FOOD JOURNAL

- Go old school and just write things down in a notebook.
- Use this food database to find the calorie & macronutrient information of any food: nutritiondata.self.com

OPTION #2—FOOD TRACKING SOFTWARE & APPS

- Keep track on your computer or smartphone. I suggest the My Fitness Pal app: www.myfitnesspal.com

Step #11—Make Subtle Adjustments at Sticking Points

So you are tracking your food intake and consistently hitting your target diet numbers (and workouts), yet still not reaching your fat loss and physique goals.

And when I say "consistent," I don't mean in quick-fix fitness industry terms—consistent for seven days. I mean more like no bullshit athlete terms—seven weeks, or even seven months. Real-world results outside of marketing material, especially elite physique results, take time.

But as a committed dude or diva, let's say things have all been on fat-slashing point for a decent amount of time, and we need to make a move to get back in the physique transformation groove.

What's the next step down the 6-Pack Checklist we can try?

You might need to make some subtle adjustments to your diet numbers in order to keep things moving along (or more accurately, to keep fat moving off your body).

Subtle Cuts vs. Super (Extreme) Cuts

This is where many physique peeps get impatient and make extreme calorie and carb cuts to try to speed up the fat loss process. This can lead to a lot of physiological, metabolic, and hormonal drawbacks and set the dieter up for huge body fat rebounds and yo-yo roller coaster rides.

The better play call is to make subtle, non-extreme adjustments to your initial program.

More specifically, if you are eating at 12 cals/lb of lean body mass or target bodyweight, drop it down to a reasonable 11 cals/lb for a month or two, and re-assess from there. Or if you think in terms of percentages, drop your calories by 5-15% and see what happens. More drastic shifts are usually unnecessary.

What you don't want to do is cut your calories in half and carbs to zero, thinking you can starve your way to a 6-pack. It sounds crazy, but a lot of people do it and end up suffering the consequences of following such extreme plans.

And quite honestly, these are already pretty aggressive fat loss diet numbers. If you can't get lean eating at the low end of 10 cals/lb of lean body mass or target bodyweight, you should probably consult with a physician to rule out any underlying medical condition (metabolic, hormonal, genetic, etc.), or to see if you need a medically supervised plan.

Miyaki's Preferred Method: Make Subtle Calorie Adjustments via Shifts in Carbohydrate Intake

1. Given a healthy, active demographic that strength trains three or more times a week, I generally recommend keeping protein and dietary fat relatively constant regardless of the diet phase.
2. You always want to set protein at optimal levels for muscle growth, or at least maintenance.
3. You want to provide a baseline level of essential fatty acids and good fats for natural hormone production and other health benefits (getting the majority of that fat primarily as a by-product of your protein foods).
4. You also want to keep some veggies, fruits, and/or roots in your diet for micronutrients, phytonutrients, fiber, and satiety.

5. The only thing left to adjust is your starchy carbohydrate intake. So you simply adjust the calories and starchy carbs up or down based on your current goals. If you want to lose more fat, carbs come down. If you are losing weight too fast (a sign of muscle loss) or want to shift your focus to gaining muscle, carbs go up.

Step #12—Integrate Carb Refeeds When Lean

Hopefully you understand by now that to burn off stored body fat and unveil your 6-pack, you must take in fewer calories than you expend, on average, over some time frame.

Did you see the subtle takeaway there? You must *average* a calorie deficit over some time frame. The most common way is through a consistent daily deficit.

Linear Diet Plans

For most people, starting out on the road to dropping body fat and looking phenomenal with your shirt off, pants off, or walking around naked is simple.

Well, at least from the waist up and the quads down. That nether region in between might require a pair of fancy clippers and complex trimming methods. I know how to navigate my own home zones. But quite frankly, yours are a personal problem beyond my expertise. You must learn to solve that riddle for yourself.

But back to the lesson at hand and our fat-slashing game plan. For beginners, it is pretty straightforward. Girl or dude, you are probably just eating way too much refined and fast food. Clean it up, control your portions, get in that damn calorie deficit necessary for fat loss, and frickin' stay there on a daily basis.

Have one or two cheat meals a week for flexibility and sustainability (no one is going to cut out the crappy foods we love indefinitely) and for social reasons (I usually recommend saving those meals for the weekend when you are out and about and don't want to obsess about your diet like a crazy person).

Or, eat rock solid during the week when you are in work/get-stuff-done mode anyway, and then loosen up a little on the weekends. This does not mean trying to beat Kobayashi in a hot dog eating contest. Simply eat reasonable portions of some of the foods you love.

If you are over 15-20% body fat, the pregame pep talk is over. Stop analyzing. Start doing. Don't overcomplicate things or confuse yourself with more advanced protocols. Clean it up, be consistent, and start moving in the right direction.

Linear Diet Problems

The leaner you become (under 15-20%), however, the more detailed and strategic you need to get. But I don't want to give the impression after the last section that the final 6-pack answer is to just keep cutting your calories and carbs down to zero.

There definitely comes a point of diminishing returns with calorie cuts, and you may need to integrate a more advanced strategy to get the final body fat-slashing job done.

You might need to use some type of cyclical plan to make your final fat loss stand. Why?

A straight up linear method to dieting, where you just continue cutting calories until you reach your goals, rarely works in taking you all the way home to the 6-Pack Zone.

And if it does, it often leads to huge weight rebounds when you return to more normal/maintenance calorie levels. You know, after you've suffered through some extreme dieting phase to get a photo to trick people on your e-dating website profile page.

You see, the human body is a highly adaptive organism and eventually adapts to any calorie deficit. The net effect is that the longer and more consistently you diet, the harder it becomes to continue getting results, and the more likely it is that you will hit a plateau.

This is related to a hormone called leptin, which downregulates during caloric restriction. Reduced leptin levels increase hunger and cravings while slowing the metabolic rate and reducing energy expenditure—not a good combo for slashing stubborn fat.

In addition, leptin is a master control hormone, meaning its levels can impact other hormones. During prolonged calorie deficits, levels of testosterone, growth hormone, IGF-1, and thyroid can all drop.

This combination can lead to muscle loss and the inability to drop those pesky last few layers of body fat that are holding on for dear life.

We conclude that there are significant differences between men and women in the responses of leptin (36% drop for men, 61% drop for women) and insulin to 7 days of energy restriction.

Dubuc et al. **Changes of serum leptin and endocrine and metabolic parameters after 7 days of energy restriction in men and women.** Metabolism. 1998 Apr;47(4):429-34.

From the *European Journal of Endocrinology*:

More and more data are emerging that leptin is not only important in the regulation of food intake and energy balance, but that it also has a function as a metabolic and neuroendocrine hormone . . . Leptin itself exerts effects on different endocrine axes, mainly on the hypothalamic-pituitary-gonadal axis and on insulin metabolism, but also on the hypothalamic-pituitary-adrenal, thyroid and GH axes. Leptin may thus be considered a new endocrine mediator, besides its obvious role in body weight regulation.

The Calorie Boost Solution

Periodic overfeeding—or a couple of days of calorie surpluses sprinkled in among days of calorie deficits—can offset some of the negative effects of chronic caloric restriction.

A day or two of refeeding can boost leptin, testosterone, thyroid, and growth hormone to normal, prediet levels. It can resensitize the body to the fat loss process and help you break through a plateau.

Due to restocked glycogen stores, it can also ramp up lagging training intensity and enthusiasm that can slowly set in during prolonged calorie deficits.

It sounds completely counterintuitive, but I've had clients lose two pounds the next week after a day of jacking up calories and carbs.

Despite a weight loss of only 2.6 +/- 0.8%, mean plasma leptin levels fell by 61.9 +/- 25.2% (8.5 +/- 4.5 to 2.4 +/- 0.5 ng/mL, P < 0.01) in 7 nonobese females subjected to 3 days of fasting. Leptin levels in fasted subjects returned to baseline within 12 h of refeeding.

Weigle, et al. **Effect of fasting, refeeding, and dietary fat restriction on plasma leptin levels.** J Clin Endocrinol Metab. 1997 Feb;82(2):561-5.

From the *International Journal of Obesity and Related Metabolic Disorders*:

CHO OF (carbohydrate overfeeding) increased plasma leptin concentrations by 28%, and 24 h EE by 7%. FAT OF (fat overfeeding) did not significantly change plasma leptin concentrations or energy expenditure.

There are many cyclical dieting strategies that can work well. And as you can see, carbohydrates impact leptin levels more so than dietary fat, so they often involve manipulating carbohydrate intake for maximum fat-burning effects.

Miyaki's Preferred Method: The 5-2 Carb Refeed Plan

1. 5-6 days a week eat your base fat loss diet (10-13 calories per/lb). This includes training and non-training days.
2. 1-2 days a week spike calories to maintenance levels or higher (15+).
3. Since carbohydrates increase leptin levels more so than dietary fats or protein, I recommend increasing calories

primarily via carbohydrates (carb loading, carb refeeding, or whatever else you crazy kids are calling it these days).
4. In other words, protein and dietary fat remain relatively the same throughout the week. Carbs go up or down based on the day.

More Extreme Carb Cycling Plans

Technically, the above plan is a carb-cycling plan because protein and fat remain constant, and calories go up or down via carbohydrates.

Some coaches recommend more extreme fluctuations in carbs, with an accompanying increase or decrease in dietary fat to compensate. This is what some would consider true carb cycling. Here's how that looks with a relatively normal/sane training program:

- On rest days (3-4 days a week), eat a lower calorie and carbohydrate diet with carbs coming primarily from vegetables and whole fruits. No starches. Make up the rest of your calorie requirements with dietary fat (fattier cuts of meat and/or added whole food fats).
- On training days (3-4 days a week), eat a higher calorie and carbohydrate diet. Get your dietary fat as a by-product of relatively lean protein sources, don't add fats, and get the rest of your calorie requirements from starchy carbohydrates.

If this works well for you, great, do it. There is a lot of flexibility with how you average your calorie deficit, and manage your maintenance of a normal metabolic rate and natural hormone production.

But there are a few reasons why I prefer my 5-2 Refeed Route, with less extreme fluctuations in daily carbohydrate intake, and including some starchy carbs even on off days from training.

Daily Carbs & Baseline Brain Function

If in a non-ketogenic adapted state (which I don't think is necessary, nor optimal, for higher-level physique goals), you still need about 100-150g of carbs a day to support liver glycogen reserves, normal blood sugar, and brain and CNS functioning.

It is true that once muscle glycogen stores are high, they will stay high until intense training is performed. But since liver glycogen is used to regulate normal blood sugar, it can become depleted on a daily basis, even without training.

Thus, going no carb on off days can cause some to experience symptoms such as low energy, poor cognitive function, irritability, and foul mood. Perhaps that's why there are so many people in the fitness industry who seem to be miserable, pissed off, and emotionally disturbed all of the time.

So to stay a cool dude or girl, I recommend keeping a baseline level of carbs in your diet, even on off days.

Daily Carbs & Refueling From Intense Training

Glycogen restoration can take 24 hours or more. So on your rest days, you are still restocking glycogen stores that you depleted through intense training sessions.

This is especially true if you are operating in a slight calorie deficit and are only eating a modest amount of daily carbs in order to slash fat or maintain a ripped physique.

In a depleted state, carbs will be used to restock glycogen stores first before spilling over into fat stores. Yes, even on off days.

It's like this. Let's say you drove your car around all day and hit "E" (an intense workout), yet only had enough cash to put a quarter of a tank of gas back in that night (moderate calorie and carb deficits).

The next day you don't have to drive your car (off day), but the day after that, you have to take a road trip (another intense workout). At some point before that trip, you'll have to hit the gas station again and put in a little more fuel for the road (some carbs on off days).

Even if you put in another quarter or even half a tank of gas on that off day, you'll never hit "Full" or have any spill over the sides (fat gain). Yet you'll have enough gas to drive around every day (proper fuel for your workouts).

Damn, I don't know if that makes sense to you, but I'm doing my best. It makes sense to me, but I'm a little off.

Daily Carbs & Proper Preworkout Fuel

Keep in mind that the meals on your off days from training are part of your pre-workout fuel for you next day's training.

Like I said, it is true that once muscle glycogen stores are full, they will stay full until intense training is performed. So theoretically, you could reload your muscle glycogen stores after an intense workout, eat no carbs the next day or two off from the gym, and have plenty of muscle glycogen stores whenever you do hit it again.

However, depleted muscle glycogen stores are generally not the limiting factor in diets that include some carbs, either daily or in cycling style.

It is liver glycogen that normalizes blood sugar and provides fuel for the brain and central nervous system both at rest and during activity. And the rate at which the body burns liver glycogen stores during intense training can increase up to ten times.

You don't have to worry about da geek stuff, but just realize that depleted liver glycogen stores are what generally cause symptoms of low blood sugar, full body and central nervous system fatigue, and impaired performance in the gym.

And again, since liver glycogen stores are small and are used even at rest, they can become depleted on a daily basis. So some carbs, even on off days, are necessary to restock liver glycogen stores and provide proper fuel for your next day's workouts.

Maybe these smart guys can better clarify it for you:

> *In prolonged, intense exercise, blood glucose eventually falls below normal levels because liver glycogen depletes and active muscles continue to use the available blood glucose. Symptoms of an abnormally reduced blood glucose or hypoglycemia include weakness, hunger, and dizziness. Reduced blood glucose ultimately impairs exercise performance and partially explains "central" fatigue associated with prolonged exercise.*
> —McArdle and Katch, *Sport and Exercise Nutrition*

Daily Carbs & Preventing Muscle Loss

Catabolic activity and the use of amino acids as fuel are greatest when trying to perform strength training or other forms of anaerobic training in a liver glycogen–depleted state.

The body's number one priority at all times is to provide fuel for the brain and central nervous system, not to build or even maintain lean muscle mass.

If you perform anaerobic training with depleted liver glycogen stores, the body will still find a way to provide fuel for the brain. It will break down amino acids from muscle tissue and convert them to glucose. This is a catabolic activity that, if repeated chronically, will lead to muscle loss.

So some carbs on your off days from training may prevent losing muscle during your next day's training session.

The basic summary is if you're training three or more days a week, everything that you eat matters, not just what you eat on training days. All meals are either part of your post-workout or pre-workout nutrition.

One more check in with Da Geeks (and as a fellow geek, I mean that with the highest respect):

> *Protein use for energy reaches its highest level during exercise in a glycogen-depleted state. This emphasizes the important role carbohydrate plays as a protein sparer. It further indicates that carbohydrate availability inhibits protein catabolism in exercise.*
> —McArdle and Katch, *Sport and Exercise Nutrition*

Daily Carbs & Consistent Sleep

One of the most overlooked steps for optimal fat loss is quality sleep. This is where the majority of our repair and recovery processes take place. It's also the critical time of the day where we get the biggest spike in our most potent fat-burning hormone—growth hormone.

If you don't get consistent sleep, you won't maximally burn body fat.

Carbs trigger serotonin release, which relaxes us and induces sleep. Many athletes who train hard and try to cut carbs at night complain of insomnia.

One of the biggest complaints I consistently hear about more extreme carb-cycling protocols is that on the "high" days, sleep is great. But on the "low" days, sleep sucks. One day you're wet dreaming, and the next day you're trying to avoid having a Nightmare on Elm Street.

Why not evenly distribute your carbs over two days so you can catch some solid sack time every night?

Instead of going with the extreme high of 400g of carbs on training days and the extreme lows of 0g on off days, why not go with a more moderate approach of 150-200g of carbs on baseline days, with a few refeeds of 300g or so?

Calorie & Carb Cycling Conclusions

My preferred plan is to spend most of the week in a slight calorie deficit (five to six days a week), with one to two carb refeed days. Many physique competitors and fitness models use this approach with great success.

More extreme carb cycling can definitely work, and if you feel great on that plan, keep sticking to it. But I don't think it's necessary for optimum results. There are a variety of ways you can structure your diet and reach the same end goal; the key is finding what makes your plan the easiest to follow in the real world.

I'm a daily deficit and refeed guy.

You?

Try both approaches out and stick with whatever works best. I don't really give a damn what you settle on as a plan. I just want you to find something that works great for you.

SECTION III
OUTRO

6-Pack Checklist Summary

We've covered a lot in this book. So to make sure that all translates into some simple, straightforward, and actionable strategies you can apply to reach your goals, let's summarize it in an "Official" 6-Pack Checklist.

1. Get in the calorie deficit necessary for fat loss (10-13 calories/lb of lean body mass or target bodyweight).
2. Cut back on refined, processed, and hyperpalatable foods.
3. Emphasize predominantly high satiety whole foods (the island-style diet is a decent template: animal proteins, whole fruit, root vegetables, vegetables, and white rice).
4. Eat optimum levels of protein (0.7-0.9g/lb of lean body mass or target bodyweight, rounding up to 1g/lb if you wish).
5. Strength train a few times a week with hypertrophy parameters.
6. Keep dietary fat intake moderate in order to leave some room for carbs (0.2-0.33g/lb of lean body mass or target bodyweight).
7. Fill in all remaining calories with carbohydrates. This will likely fall in the range of 1-2g/lb of lean body mass or target bodyweight.

8. Use whatever diet structure makes sticking to your plan as practical, functional, and sustainable as possible. My suggested starting point is the 3 & Feast Strategy: Eat 3 protein-based meals a day—the traditional breakfast, lunch, and dinner. Escalate your carb intake, and eat the highest percentage of your calories and carbs at night. Keep your daytime meals to a carb:pro ratio of 1:1 or less.
9. Add some non-exercise-specific physical activity (NEPA) if necessary. Start with a 30-60 minute walk on your off days.
10. Track your food intake, calories, and macronutrients if you are having trouble making progress or if you want to ramp it up to reach your peak. I recommend MyFitnessPal.
11. Make subtle adjustments if/when you hit a sticking point. Start by reducing calories by 1cal/lb of lean body mass or target weight, or 5-15% of calories. The reduction should come primarily via carbohydrates.
12. Integrate calorie spikes/carb refeeds when lean. My preferred method is a 5-2 Plan. Five to six days a week eat your base fat loss diet (10-13 calories per/lb). This includes training and non-training days. One to two days a week, spike calories to maintenance levels or higher (15+) primarily via increasing carbs.

The Final Fat-Slashing Strategy

> *Knowing is not enough; we must apply. Willing is not enough; we must do.*
> –Bruce Lee

> *When you understand what I am telling you, apply what you have learned to your everyday life . . . I am not interested with your talk about my ideas. I am more interested in your applying them to your life.*
> –Miyamoto Musashi

I want to leave you now with perhaps the most important tip of all.

The strategies I presented in this book are just the starting point. You have to get into the game and apply them in order reach your physique goals. No game in the history of mankind has ever been won by sitting on the sidelines of life and doing nothing.

Always remember that it is not what you read, think, analyze, plan, calculate, or talk about in this world that gives you results. It is all about what you DO.

Execution is everything in the end, my new fat loss friend. It doesn't matter how much knowledge you can acquire. If you are not taking action and applying it, it is all useless.

So get out there and start attacking your goals today, not tomorrow, or some other time down the line. "Some other time" usually ends up being never.

Thank You

Thanks for checking out this book. I hope the strategies within it help you get started with an effective, efficient, and sustainable fat loss plan.

This book is just the tip of the iceberg in terms of physique transformation strategies. If you dug (digged?) it and would like to learn more about any of the individual topics, I invite you to check out my book catalog on Amazon.

www.amazon.com/Nate-Miyaki/e/B005X0QSX0

From the physique-focused fitness stuff to the philosophy and lifestyle strategies, I hope you find something that helps you along your way. And I have several books in the works, so stay tuned. While your waistline is shrinking, the catalog will be expanding.

And don't forget, you can sign up to receive all of my future books for free here: natemiyaki.com/freebook

Please Leave a Short Review

If you found this book to be valuable, I ask two small favors:
1. Give me a virtual high five, kiss, or bro-hug right now. Spread the love, baby. Don't be shy.
2. Please take a quick moment to leave a review for this book on Amazon. Total transparency and honesty here—reviews really help get our books higher up in the Amazon rankings (via some Matrix-like algorithm).

This selfless and heroic act by you will help a small-timer like me get discovered by folks who can use the information the most. We also want future readers who find the work we do to be able to make an informed purchasing decision and to know that this book is different from the rest of the "Get Fit Quick" BS that exists and dominates fitness lists.

The feedback will also help me to continue getting better and to write the type of books that will ultimately help you reach your goals.

Until our paths cross again, take care, my friend.

Other Books by Nate Miyaki

Fitness Books

- *The Truth about Carbs: How to Eat Just the Right Amount of Carbs to Slash Fat, Look Great Naked, & Live Lean Year-Round*
- *The Truth about Weight Loss*
- *The Samurai Diet: The Science & Strategy of Winning the Fat Loss War*

Strategy Books

- *Rise Above*
- *A Philtered Soul*
- *The Way of the Cancer Warrior: 34 Strategies For Your Cancer War* (Free Downloadable PDF edition)

Resources

1. Jaminet, Paul. *The Perfect Health Diet.* New York, NY: Scribner, 2012
2. Cordain, Loren. *The Paleo Diet.* Hoboken, New Jersey: John Wiley & Sons, Inc. 2002
3. McArdle, William et al. *Sports and Exercise Nutrition, Third Edition.* Baltimore, MD: Lippincott Williams & Wilkins, 2008.
4. Gropper, Sareen et al. *Advanced Nutrition and Human Metabolism, Fifth Edition.* Belmont, CA: Wadsworth, Cengage Learning, 2009.
5. Jeukendrup, Asker. *Sport Nutrition, Second Edition.* Champaign, Il: Human Kinetics, Inc., 2010.
6. Whitten, Ari et al. *The Low Carb Myth.* Archangel Ink, 2015
7. Baechle, et al. *Essentials of Strength & Conditioning.* Champaign, Il: Human Kinetics Inc., 2008.
8. Aceto, Chris. *Championship Bodybuilding.* Kearney, NE: Morris Publishing, 2003.
9. Hofmekler, Ori. *The Warrior Diet.* Berkeley, CA: Blue Snake Books, 2007.
10. Aragon, Alan. *The Alan Aragon Research Review.*
11. Guyenet, Stephan. *Whole Health Source.*
12. Lee, Bruce. *Striking Thoughts: Bruce Lee's Wisdom for Daily Living.* Compiled and Edited by John Little. North Clarendon, VT: Tuttle Publishing, 2000.
13. Tsunetomo, Yamamoto. *Hagakure: The Book of the Samurai.* Bunkyo-ku, Tokyo: Kodansha International, 2002.

14. Musashi, Miyamoto. *The Book of Five Rings*. Translation by William Scott Wilson. Boston, Massachusetts: Shambhala Publications, Inc., 2002.

About the Author

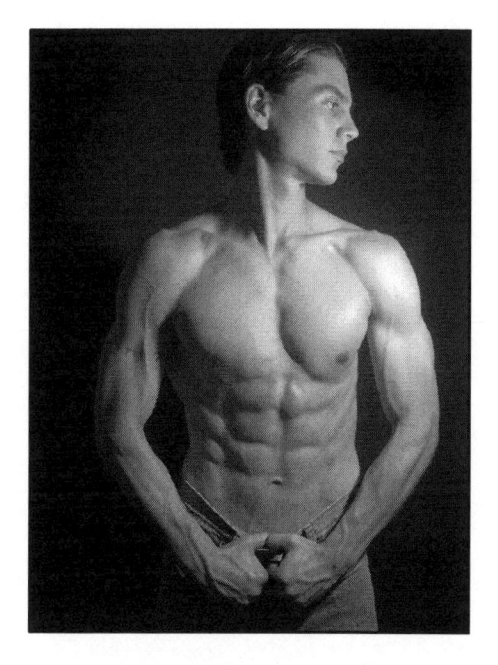

Nate Miyaki is an author, athlete, and public speaker. He has been featured in *The Huffington Post, Men's Fitness, Men's Health, Shape, Muscle & Fitness, Livestrong,* and *Paleo Fx*.

He is a two-time natural bodybuilding champion and has worked as a fitness model and representative for several fitness brands.

He speaks for corporate wellness programs, at health and fitness seminars, and consults privately with clients, ranging from pro athletes to busy professionals and entrepreneurs. He maintains a fitness, philosophy, and motivational blog at: NateMiyaki.com.

He was born and raised in the San Francisco Bay Area and graduated from the University of California, Berkeley.

And yes, he wrote this bio in the third person in hopes that it convinces you that he is way more important than he actually is!

Printed in Great Britain
by Amazon